W9-AFC-567

THE POSTURE PAIN FIX

How to fix your back, neck and other postural problems that cause pain in your body

Rosalind Ferry

Withdrawn
from the
MATC Library

LIBRARY
MILWAUKEE AREA
TECHNICAL COLLEGE
NORTH CAMPUS
5555 West Highland Road
Mequon, Wisconsin 53092

LT156
F399
2011

The Posture Pain Fix
www.rosalindferry.com
Printed in the United States
Available in Kindle on Amazon
© Rosalind Ferry, 2011

Illustrations by Elysabeth Barnett

ISBN: 978-1517513412

All rights reserved. No part of this publication pay be reproduced, stored in a retrieval system or transmitted in any form or by any means of electronic, mechanical, photocopying, recording or otherwise, without prior written permission of the author.

Always check with a health care professional before beginning any exercise program. Enlist the help of a physiotherapist for minor problems before they become bigger ones.

The information in this book is true and complete to the best of my knowledge. All recommendations are made without guarantee on the part of the author. The author disclaims all liability in connection with the use of this information.

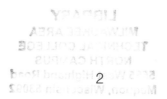

DIRECTORY

Section 3 - Correct and incorrect postures and habits 53

For Matthew and William

ACKNOWLEDGEMENTS

Various people have helped with this book, including the many patients I have treated in my physiotherapy practice over the years.

I would especially like to thank my inspirational sister-in-law, Toronto artist Elysabeth Barnett, who created its lively diagrams, and worked tirelessly to breathe life into the project.

Many thanks go to Vancouver engineer Frances Caton who helped edit the book -- and to Jon, my husband, son William and daughter-in-law Robin, who helped write, shape and organize it.

Thanks are also due to North Vancouver ergonomic physiotherapist Carmel Murphy for her invaluable input, to librarian Deb Monkman, of the Physiotherapy Association of B.C., for her patient help . . . and to my physio colleagues Susy Carnaghan, a long-time loyal friend, and Anniken Chadwick for all their suggestions.

I would like to acknowledge the advice of Alexander Technique teacher Beatty Leadbetter and other members of the Leadbetter family -- Nicky, Gordon, Louise, Ben and Claudi.

My courageous parents, Pat and Leslie, deserve enormous credit for making the book possible by never ceasing to encourage my love of Africa, animals and the outdoors.

My gorgeous grandchildren Georgia and Julian who never stopped reminding me of the balance we are all born with, but all too often lose along the way.

Last, but by no means least, I would like to thank all the horses whose boundless energy, limitless spirit and beautiful movement have given me at least some insight into nature and the natural movement that we health professionals should always try to preserve and enhance.

CODES

Ouches

The location of the "ouches" on the diagrams indicate possible problem areas on your body. These points are where muscles may be strained and joints and nerves compressed -- leading to aches and pains and increased wear and tear. I hope that, by drawing your attention to these areas, it will make you more aware of your positions and habits throughout your day.

 Possible areas of injury / pain

 Compression of vertebrae

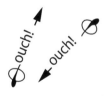 Possible pain resulting from compression of the vertebrae

 Special attention

 Watch out

9

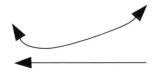

Direction of movement

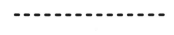

Angles of the body or parts of the body

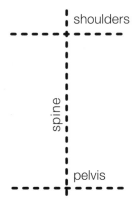

shoulders

spine

pelvis

Pay attention to **the H line.**

In the diagrams in this book, we have drawn dotted lines to help you align your shoulders and pelvis with your spine.

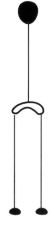

Feet hip distance apart.
See page 39.

INTRODUCTION

There is nothing more wonderful for some of us than watching a horse galloping in a field, a deer jumping over a fence or a cat moving stealthily on the hunt. It reminds us how agile and strong these creatures have remained through time. Their movements are fluid and seemingly effortless.

The same is true if you have ever seen Masai warriors walking tall, proud and effortlessly, as I did as a child growing up in Africa. They would gaze confidently out into the distance for any sign of lion or other wildlife.

Contrast this with the typical urban human ... awkward, hunched and uncoordinated. It's pretty obvious that, when it comes to ease and fluidity of movement, something has gone terribly wrong.

Too much time spent cramped over computers, clutching telephones or sitting in front of the TV has caused us to lose the healthy ways of moving of the hunter-gatherers of old. We've become tense, stressed and estranged from our own bodies ... literally uncomfortable in our own skin. Work stress, trauma, depression and domestic tension eat away at our psyche. Also, the way we move plays a huge role in how our body functions. Poor posture, our natural one-sidedness, obesity and bad habits contribute to excessive wear and tear on our joints, discs, muscles and nervous system.

Our bodies rebel, as is clear from the pain we often feel in our neck, back or shoulders. It's time we listened to what our bodies are telling us, and took notice. We should really change our habits and positions, and try to recapture the proud and efficient movement we once had.

In this book, you will learn how to develop better posture and avoid unnecessary wear and tear on your joints and discs. Through these pages of basic positions and simple exercises, you will be able to realign your body so it will function more efficiently, thereby helping eliminate aches and pains.

The book is divided into four parts:

    1. A brief description of anatomy, function and posture.

    2. Examples of incorrect and correct body positions.

    3. Some simple exercises that can be done throughout the day.

    4. Miscellaneous - tips, references and resources.

This book aims to preserve and enhance your movement and balance. It will help you identify faulty postural habits and replace them with correct ones. As a result, you will radiate new-found energy and health.

OUR ANCESTORS

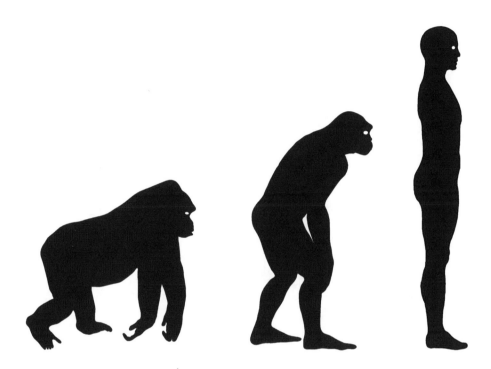

Our predecessors, the apes, have the advantage of moving around on all four limbs. This gives them a wider base on which to balance. Humans, however, have only two feet, and therefore a narrower base. This makes us less stable and affords less room for our upper body to move in and out of balance. If we allow gravity to pull us down or we wander around in a state of fight or flight, we have already compromised our ability to remain upright with ease. Therefore, we should start and continue our quest to bring our body into balance.

Our fight, flight or freeze response is there to protect us from danger. Now that we are more civilized and socialized, we also have to cope with multiple threats to our emotional and physical well-being.

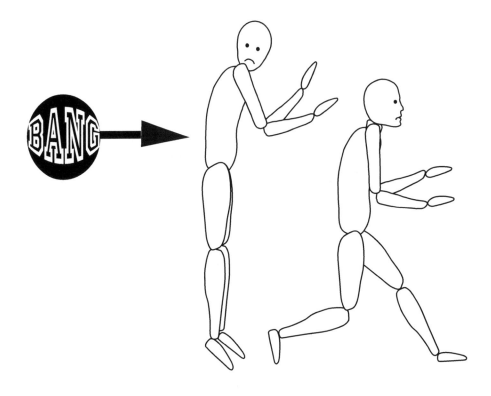

Due to this stress, this response is switched on a great deal of the time. Adrenalin is released, our shoulders go up, our neck shortens, the heart pumps faster, blood pressure goes up and we remain in a persistent state of alertness. This can put severe strain on our entire physiological system and harm our long-term way of going.

MODERN LIFE

The World Health Organization states that health is not only the absence of disease, but a complete state of mental, physical and social well-being.

Modern living is playing havoc with our bodies. According to a recent article in the Journal of the American Medical Association, low back pain is the second most common cause of disability among American adults and a common reason for lost days. More than 80 per cent of the population will experience low back pain at some point in their lives [1]. We are too sedentary and rely too much on cars, computers and other labour-saving devices. Our upper bodies are being over-used, while our lower bodies are heavily under-utilized and our spines are taking the stress. There is also a cultural preference in the west for upper-body strength.

Our connection to people and the natural world around us has changed. We no longer stand tall and erect or walk freely and relaxedly with loose limbs. We crouch over our computers and hunch up our shoulders while in rapt attention to our hand-held devices. We need to move more and sit less.

We are living longer. But we rely more on costly surgical operations to keep us moving and replace our worn-out hips and knee joints. Certainly, these operations can rid us of our pain. But they are not without risks, including the risk that we become dependent on the surgeon's knife to fix our physical problems rather than putting our bodies in a position to heal by themselves.

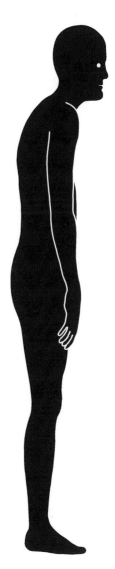

The American Physical Therapy Association noted recently that, according to a study published in the New England Journal of Medicine, physical therapy combined with comprehensive medical management was just as effective as surgery at relieving the pain and stiffness of moderate to severe osteoarthritis of the knee [2].

Also, public health costs are rising at an alarming rate. And a consensus is emerging among politicians, health administrators and medical practitioners that it is both healthier and more cost-effective for people to learn to take care of their own bodies -- and to leave surgeries for emergencies and other special situations.

I always remember one of my elderly male patients, whose body was rapidly deteriorating, telling me that, if only he had known he would live this long, he would have taken better care of himself.

HABITS

Old Habits

We all have habits, some of which we are aware and many of which we are not. Consciously or unconsciously, we fail to live in the moment. We tend to think about the future or the past, not the present. And therefore we become unaware of our current tensions and the resulting unnatural positions in which we constantly place our bodies. Eventually, these fixed and habitual patterns restrict our natural movement, and our way of going becomes laboured. This not only slows us down physically, but fatigues us mentally.

According to the National Health Service (NHS), it is estimated that 1 in 5 people in Britain visited their GP each year complaining of back pain [3]. The NHS also explains that "how you sit, stand and lie down can have a important effect on your back" [4].

New Habits

Developing more efficient ways of moving is not easy. There is no quick fix to poor physical habits learned over a lifetime. You will have to practise many times to open up fresh neural pathways, so that new habits become normal and old ones feel foreign and able to be discarded.

Over the years, my efforts to become a better horse rider foundered because of physical limitations I had unknowingly placed on myself. I tended to blame shortcomings in the horse for our poor performances in the dressage arena. It was only later in life that I realized it was my tensions and imbalances that were inhibiting the horse and stifling its movement. I was forced to go back to the basics of training, including relaxation, awareness, balance and the development of good posture. Only then could my horse move more freely and become more balanced -- as nature intended.

The Brain

The brain is the powerhouse. To increase self awareness and conscious movement, the brain has to be trained to master this skill.

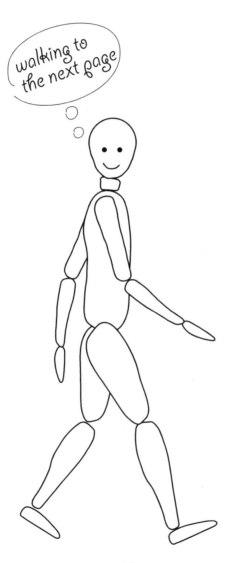

SECTION 1

Principles of Good Posture

EQUILIBRIUM

To function properly, the human body needs to have a balance between flexibility, strength, mobility, relaxation, an uncluttered mind and conscious movement. With all our responsibilities, family, jobs and stress, this natural equilibrium is mostly lost. **Slow Down, You Move Too Fast** is a great song and an even better motto.

We are born with the capacity to be fluid and adaptive. During our early life, we enjoy a wide range of motion in our joints. We can walk on such uneven surfaces as rocks, sand and mud. And we can sit almost anywhere, on the floor or on a rock. We can float or swim, run, jump, climb, roll, bend down, stretch up, reach sideways and backwards. We can look up to the sky or down at the ground as well as twist this way and that.

We need muscular strength to support our skeletons, protect our joints and help us push, pull and lift. We also need to know how to move our body parts to minimize the risk of injury and eventual breakdown of our bodies.

A clear mind and a relaxed, aware approach are the way to prolong mobility and reduce wear and tear. Unfortunately, after years of walking on flat, hard surfaces and sitting in chairs in poor positions, we are wearing out rapidly. Our lives are geared to mechanical devices that do most activities for us. Then, we go to the gym and exercise by pulling and pushing our arms and legs against an unyielding resistance. We rarely extend our range of movement by using our limbs freely.

Our amazing human adaptability has allowed us to adjust to compromised body movement and function. Too many of us accept our limitations as inevitable, and deterioration is the obvious result. To a large extent, age is not the issue here. My father who is 87 can still fully squat to do his gardening. He has been doing this throughout his adult life.

If you allow your bodily health to wear down, you will find that you wind up falling as you get older. Older adults are hospitalized five times more for fall-related injuries than any other group.

Exercises / activities

Temperament plays a large part in the choice of our activities. Some people prefer soft, gentle workouts, others prefer harder, more fiery ones. Whichever one you choose, bear in mind that the activity needs to be balanced -- so that you body is not strained in any one direction.

Yoga and martial arts are good disciplines to follow. Tai Chi is a 5,000 year old Chinese discipline and helps to prolong life, build strength, stamina, concentration, balance and flexibility. You could also check out Qigong qi-(chi) life energy. This is a practice of aligning the body, breath and mind for health, meditation and martial arts training. Pilates, the Alexander Technique and the Feldenkrais Method are also highly beneficial. Sports and other recreational activities should be included. The key is to find an activity that you can enjoy, suits your body and becomes a part of your routine.

To improve your health, try envisaging the life you want to lead and start planning how you will achieve it, perhaps with the help of a knowledgeable professional. The will and desire to achieve your physical and mental goals is important. As the Latin quotation says: Mens sana in corpore sano, a healthy mind in a healthy body.

It is never too late to begin. Even 80-year-olds can benefit from an exercise regime if they begin carefully and slowly. Everyone should check with a health care professional before beginning any exercise program.

THE PAUSE

Most of us these days are so busy rushing around from one task to another that we have far too much adrenalin coursing through our bodies. We're going nowhere fast. This is not only very tiring, it is also unhealthy. We're damaging everything from our circulatory to our musculoskeletal and nervous systems. And over time, this stress can wear us down and eventually destroy us. We need to slow down and reconnect with our bodies, like the animals around us.

For example, before a cat attacks a mouse, it pauses, focuses, weighs its options and prepares to pounce. Only then does it strike, with potentially deadly power.

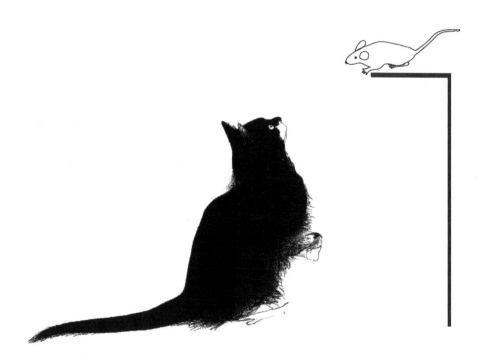

It's the same with humans who rely on timing and physical coordination to execute precise or risky manoeuvres. Whether they're soccer players about to take a penalty or professional truckers set to make a lane change, they take a moment to set themselves up for success. They pause, focus and prepare themselves for action. That is the only way they can control their bodies and environment around them. Being frantic simply doesn't cut it when you're on the prowl.

So, when I use the word "pause" in this book, it's a signal for you to slow down and take notice of your body position. Prepare yourself for action. It is only through this kind of preparation and awareness that you will be able to make a conscious change to your posture and habits. "More haste, less speed" and "look before you leap" should be your mantras.

POSTURE & AWARENESS

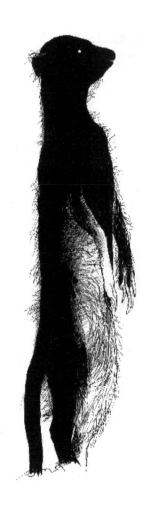

"Posture" comes from the Latin verb meaning "to put or place." It refers to the carriage of the body as a whole, whether sitting, standing or moving.

The key to good posture is to look confident and erect, but relaxed. There should be no rigidity in maintaining a good self-carriage. And for that, you could do worse than to take a tip from the Meercat. This endearing little animal from southern Africa will remind you to lengthen your neck upwards and the rest of your spine downwards while releasing your shoulders down and outwards. Now, soften your eyes and look ahead and you will begin to notice more in your peripheral vision. We are so used to looking downwards, avoiding eye contact and looking at close objects that we unbalance our spines. Our head weighs from 10 to 14 pounds. And that places a substantial burden on our neck muscles. So, if we want to reduce this muscular tension, we need to find a point of balance for the head rather like a ball on a cue stick.

BALANCE

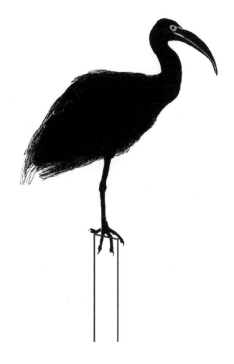

Look at the picture of the stork above, and you will see a graceful, leggy bird that seems effortlessly balanced, thanks to a system built out of millions of nerve cells.

We humans have a similar system that allows us to stand on the ground or even to remain upright on a narrow balance beam. This central nervous system and the systems associated with it work amazingly well most of the time. But an injury, an inner-ear problem, a neurological disorder, aging or poor posture can all affect our balance. That's when balance exercises and other postural training can be very beneficial in helping to correct or fine-tune this system.

See pages 152-153 for two balance exercises.

STRETCHING

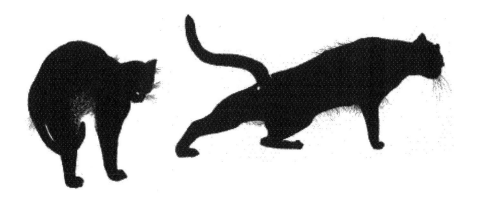

For muscles to be healthy and perform well, they need to be able to lengthen and shorten.

That is why stretching is essential, if you want to move as nature intended humans to do. Cats and other animals stretch regularly so they are ready to pounce or run. Static activities such as driving a car, sitting in front of a computer and sipping a coffee do not make for a well-oiled body. In fact, they tend to put it out of kilter and create an asymmetrical pull from the muscles around the joints, which can lead to serious wear and tear and aches and pains. Regular stretching should therefore be included in any physical activity.

MEDITATION

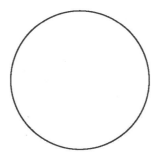

Clearing our heads is often as important as positioning our bodies. Studies have shown the merits of daily meditation [5]. It helps to combat stress, lower blood pressure and strengthen our immune system. It also helps us to sleep better. Creative visualization is another powerful meditation technique.

If you are new to meditation, you could start slowly with 10 minutes a day in a quiet area of your home. You can sit or lie down. However, focus on breathing from your belly and repeating a word or phrase as you breathe out. Your mind will be filled with many thoughts, but be persistent and you will feel amazingly refreshed.

There are many approaches to meditation. It is important to find one that suits you.

BREATHING

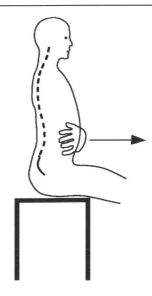

These days we tend to live hurried, breathless lives. But filling our lungs with air is as essential to basic living as it is to singing an opera. And breathing from our belly is the best way to do it. Belly breathing tells our heart and other vital organs to relax. It reduces pain, stress and blood pressure. It can also clear and focus our minds.

To breathe properly, you should use your diaphragm muscle, which creates a vacuum in your lungs to draw the air in. The muscle is positioned at the base of your rib cage. So, when it is stretched with belly breathing, it can also release tension in your back.

One good exercise is to place your hand on your belly and completely exhale. Then allow the air to fill your lungs again, without moving your back or shoulders. Once you can do this with ease, breathe in deeply to the count of four, hold your breath for seven seconds and breathe out slowly for eight. Repeat this 10 or 20 times a day. Practise this technique regularly, and you will notice the benefits. But be careful not to arch your lower and mid-back.

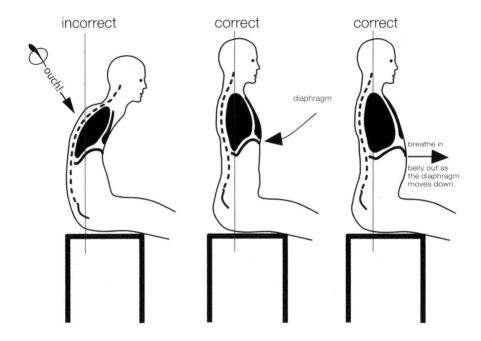

Incorrect

When sitting, if your mid-back is slumped so your upper chest is aiming downwards towards your knees, there will be less space for your diaphragm muscle to function properly. Your muscles, your ribs and spine will become tight and stiff. The result will be further unnecessary aches and pains, poor posture and decreased breathing ability.

Correct mid-back position.

Elongate the back of your neck. Then, imagine a string on the top of your head lifting you upwards, while the rest of your spine below your neck is relaxing downwards. Don't slump. Now, fill your belly with air and feel how your ribs circling your back and abdomen have more space for your lungs to breathe.

SLEEP

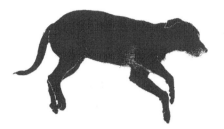

Lack of sleep causes everything from muscle aches to memory loss. It can cause poor performance at work and lead to ill health, metabolic and endocrine problems [6]. An average person needs seven to eight hours of sleep daily. Most of us do not get enough, and tend to wander around like zombies. Falling asleep at the wheel is one of the leading causes of traffic accidents as well as texting.

There are many things you can do to help yourself sleep better. Try to get into a regular sleep pattern by going to bed at the same time each night. If you can avoid it, do not sleep in on the weekend, as this will disturb your rhythm. It may take you half the week to bring it back to normal.

1. Do not eat chocolate or drink caffeinated drinks after 2 p.m.

2. Stop using the computer for at least one to two hours before bed, otherwise your mind will be in overdrive. Blue light, in particular from electronic devices, can effect the release of the hormone melatonin associated with sleep.

3. Do not eat two to three hours before going to sleep.

4. Having a warm bath, reading a book, listening to restful music or doing some relaxed breathing may help you sleep.

5. Face your alarm clock away from your field of view, so you aren't tempted to look at the time.

6. If you wake up and cannot get back to sleep, try doing something restful, but above all do not panic about the time.

7. If getting to sleep becomes an ongoing problem, seek help from your doctor or other health professional.

RELAXATION

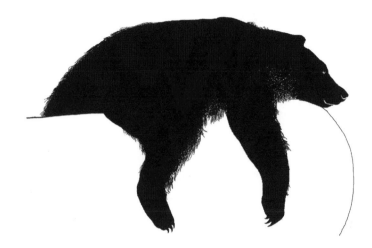

Resting relaxation

This means a release of tension and a return to equilibrium.

There are many ways to attain relaxation, including through music, meditation, sport and recreation.... or like a bear, doing very little. Learning to read your body for signs of tension and finding ways of "letting go" are important for your well-being.

Dynamic relaxation

Dynamic relaxation does not mean flopping. It can mean a quiet readiness. We need our postural muscles to hold us up against gravity, and the phasic muscles need to be ready to move our joints. Most of us, however, carry far too much unnecessary tension in our muscles. Clenching our jaws, necks, shoulders and hands while on the phone can greatly add to wear and tear on our bodies.

When learning something new, it is easy to increase tension in your body, because it is ingrained in us to try to get things right. It is much better not to worry about getting things perfect. Learning is a lifelong process. So it is best to enjoy this and be relaxed about it.

SECTION 2

Anatomy

MUSCLES - Postural and Phasic

Our **postural muscles**, which include spinal, hip flexors and calf muscles, help keep us upright against gravity. They can work for long periods, but are prone to shorten and become tight with over-use and then become painful.

Our phasic muscles are more suited to movement. They tire more easily than postural muscles, but can become inhibited and weak.

It is important to keep both muscle groups functioning well to maintain fluid joint movements and minimize musculo-skeletal imbalances.

A balanced workout combines stretching the postural muscles and strengthening the phasic muscles. This leads to greater efficiency of movement and reduces feelings of tiredness and stress.

CHILDREN

Young children naturally bend through their hips, knees and ankles. Their heads remain balanced as they learn to stand, squat, walk and run.

Unfortunately, after they start sitting in chairs, at desks, and become involved in sedentary pastimes, their achilles tendons may begin to tighten and muscular problems may develop. This can happen at around the age of six. Children often lose their natural ease of movement and begin to develop postural problems because of increasing misalignment.

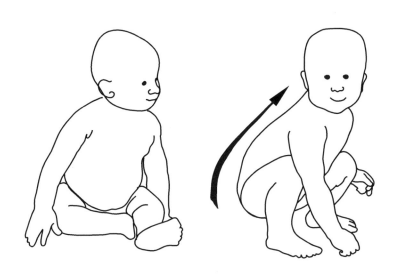

VERTEBRAE

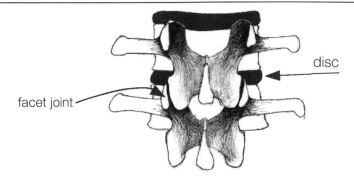

facet joint

disc

This diagram shows two vertebral bodies, with the disc in between them. The disc acts as a shock absorber or cushion. The facet joint allows movement between the two bodies so that you can bend forwards, backwards, sideways and can rotate your spine. Ligaments (fibrous tissue) connect bone to bone, creating stability between bones.

You have 7 vertebrae in your neck, 12 in your thoracic spine and 5 in your lumbar spine. Through time, these structures all develop some wear and tear. This book is intended to show you how, with increased awareness, improving posture and other minor corrections, you can reduce your aches and pains and other stress on your system.

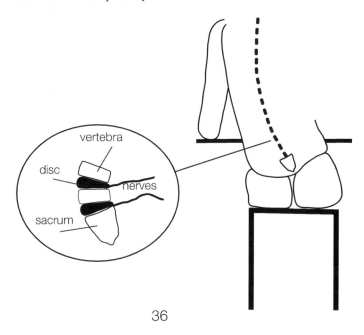

vertebra

disc

nerves

sacrum

Side view

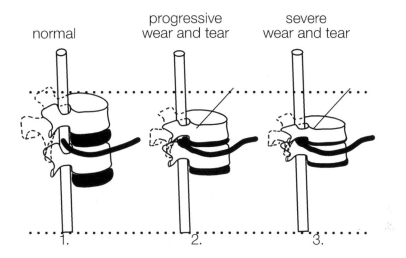

1. The first diagram shows a healthy unit: two vertebrae, the discs, the spinal cord and the black nerve root emerging from between the two vertebrae.

2. The second shows the effects of excessive loading and compression – a result of poor posture, tight muscles, trauma and bad habits.

3. The third shows narrowing where the nerve root emerges between the vertebrae. This is not good for your spine, and will give rise to nerve pressure and pain.

LUMBAR SPINE & SIT BONES

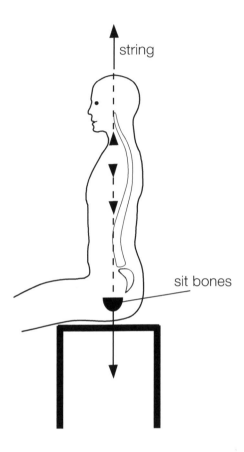

string

sit bones

Sit on a firm surface. Place your hands under your buttocks, palm side up. Feel for the bony prominences pressing into each hand. These are the sit bones. They are like little rockers. Slowly rock backwards and forwards using your hips, while keeping a straight back. Stop when you feel you are sitting at the centre point. See if you can align your shoulders over this centre point.

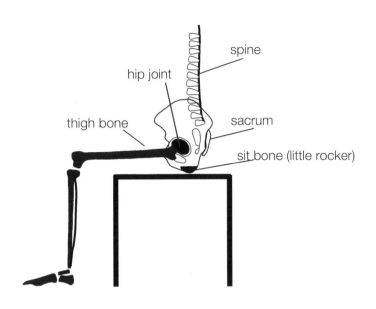

spine

hip joint

thigh bone

sacrum

sit bone (little rocker)

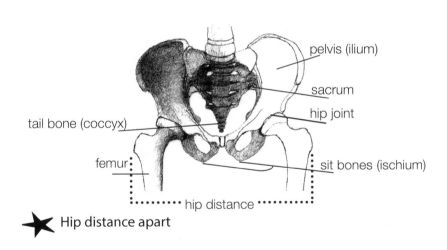

pelvis (ilium)

sacrum

hip joint

tail bone (coccyx)

femur

sit bones (ischium)

hip distance

★ Hip distance apart

THE NEUTRAL LUMBAR SPINE

INCORRECT

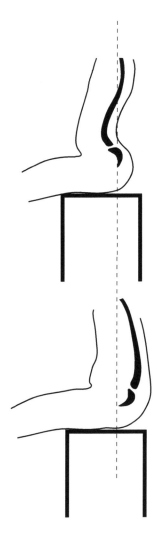

In the sitting position, fully arch or hollow your lower back, without causing pain. This is an extreme and undesirable, prolonged position.

Now, let your lower back slump and round completely, which is another extreme and undesirable, prolonged position.

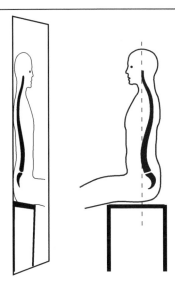

Find the half-way point between the two lumbar spine extremes, shown on the previous page. That point is your neutral position and is the desirable one. While you maintain this spinal position, line your shoulders up over your sit bones. If you are not sure you have the correct position, keep your back straight and swing forwards and backwards, using your hips as a hinge. Stop moving when your shoulders are aligned over your sit bones (see pages 38-39 for lumbar spine and sit bones).

For this exercise, it can be helpful to sit in front of a mirror, both facing it and sitting sideways, to give you feedback. Old habits may give us wrong information. We may think we are vertical when we are not.

Standing. Maintain this spinal position when standing or walking. See page 49, diagram 2 for standing and pages 64-65 for walking.

 While correcting your position, notice what your feet are doing. Try to feel their open, solid connection to the ground.

MID-BACK THORACIC POSITION AND BREATHING

INCORRECT

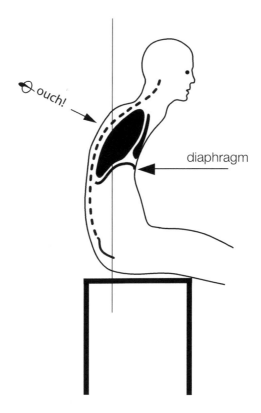

ouch!

diaphragm

While sitting, notice if your mid-back is slumped over towards your knees. If it is, you will limit the ability of the diaphragm (main breathing muscle) to work. This muscle attaches on the inside of your lower rib cage and pushes downwards and outwards as you breathe in to allow the lungs to expand. If your mid-back becomes strained through poor posture, your muscles will become tight, your ribs will stiffen and your ability to breathe fully will be limited.

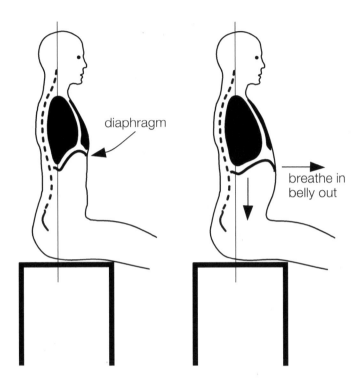

Correct mid back position.

Elongate the back of your neck while lengthening the front of your torso upwards as if you were closing a zipper from your crotch to the base of the front of your neck (page 44 & 142-143). Slowly breathe out, feeling your ribs move downwards towards your hips. Keep your shoulders relaxed. Now breathe in as though you were filling your lower torso with air (see pages 28-29).

Practise this position many times and it will become second nature.

NECK

Lengthen and release your head and neck.

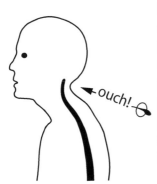

INCORRECT.
Notice how the chin is poking forward, causing too much curve in the spine. If you cup your hand around the back of your neck when you poke your chin forward, you will notice the tension in your neck muscles. This is an undesirable, prolonged position. It can cause neck and shoulder pain, headaches and even lead to arthritis.

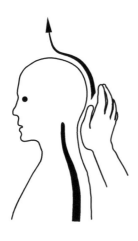

CORRECT.
With your hand still cupped around the back of your neck, bring your chin in and keep your face vertical to the wall in front. You should now feel the muscles relax. At the same time, free the **back** of your neck in an upward direction (shown by the arrow in the diagram to the left) and gap your teeth slightly to relieve any tension in your jaw. Eventually, with repetition, the freeing of the back of your neck will become your new good habit.

SHOULDERS

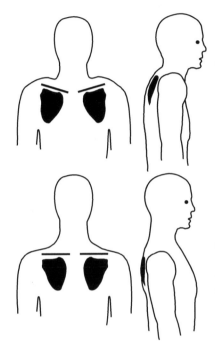

INCORRECT
Notice how the shoulders are up and rounding forward.

CORRECT
Find the correct position for your neck (as on the previous page). Also, release your shoulders back and down. Think of a downward weight dropping into your elbows. This will help with relaxation. Do not arch or round your back.

The position and relationship of your upper back and neck is critical to the mechanics of your shoulders. The shoulder is a wonderfully mobile but complex joint. It is kept stable by a set of muscles that cannot work effectively if the shoulders are hunched or rounded. This is why shoulder relaxation and proper shoulder-blade positioning are important. Correct positioning improves the mechanics of the shoulder and helps your overall body alignment.

See page 145 for a shoulder positioning exercise.

HIPS, KNEES AND FEET

In order for your hips, knees and feet to balance your body without becoming strained, you really need to pay attention to their position in certain stances.

Your back muscles maintain your upright position against gravity. Your hips, knees and ankles are meant for bending, pushing, pulling, lifting and climbing. Your quadriceps (front of your thigh), a very strong group of muscles, should be used in many day-to-day activities. You need to learn to do less with your back and more with your leg joints and thigh muscles when you bend and lift or get out of a chair. In this way, your legs will become stronger, the way nature intended.

Stand with your feet hip-distance apart so that your feet are directly under your hip joints. Bend your knees, look down at your feet and see your knees lined up over your second toes.

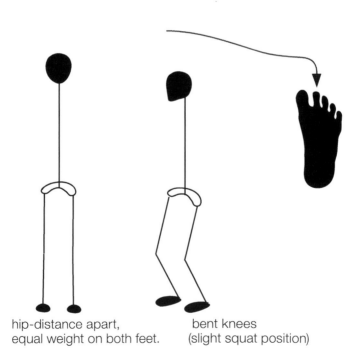

hip-distance apart,
equal weight on both feet.

bent knees
(slight squat position)

Notice if you have more weight on one foot or leg than the other. Also, as you bend, you should still be able to see your toes peeking out in front of your knees. If you cannot see them, allow your bottom to go back out behind you, as if you were preparing to sit in a chair. Don't arch your back. You can do this exercise by bending from the hips rather than the waist.

Now, feel your ankles and knees moving in their joints as you bend. When you straighten your knees and hips, feel the thrust from the muscles on the front of the thigh. When you are fully upright, make sure you can feel your ankles, knees, hips and shoulders aligning with each other.

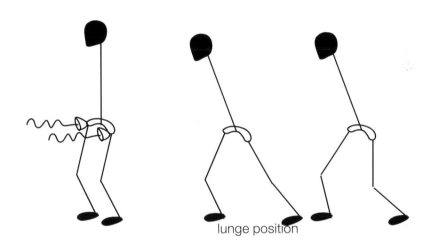

lunge position

In the lunge position (see pages 100-101. Adopted for some diagrams later in this book), place your feet hip-distance apart. Imagine you have a pair of headlights on the front of your pelvis and that the beams are shining straight ahead. Then put one leg forward in a straight line to adopt the lunge position. Make sure you feel balanced. Check the alignment of your front knee over your second toe.

You should feel no pain in any of the squat or lunge positions (see pages 146-147 for calf stretches and pages 150-151 for squat exercises). If you do, just start with a small amount of knee and hip bend, and build up your tolerance gradually.

FOOT BALANCE

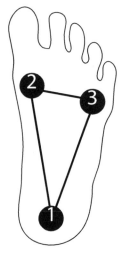

While standing, breathe in and out deeply then lower all your energy into your lower body and feet.
This will help you with your balance. Remember to do this anytime the footing is icy or unstable.

Most of us forget about our feet until they hurt. They are most important for our balance, mobility, walking and running, etc.

When you are standing, be aware of three areas on the sole of your foot:

1. The centre point of your heels
2. A point on the underside behind your big toes
3. The outside behind your little toes.

If you can, take off your shoes and socks. Rock your foot to find the centre of your heels. Then, to find the other two balance points (2 and 3), raise your toes, while keeping the rest of your feet in contact with the floor (this will raise the inside arch of your foot). Make sure you maintain equal pressure on all three points. Your feet should not tip inwards or outwards. Now, allow the toes to relax and spread wide as they resume contact with the ground. Maintain your raised arch when you do this. With regular practice this should become second nature.

Check to see if you have equal weight on each foot and between the three points. Try to do this foot-balancing exercise several times a day.

STANDING ALIGNMENT VIEWED FROM THE SIDE

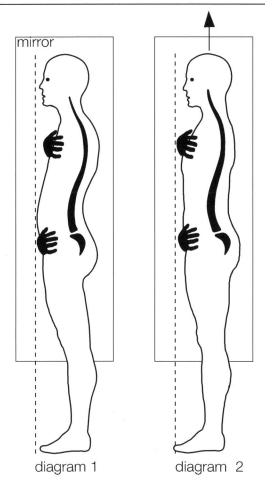

diagram 1   diagram 2

Diagram 1 shows a misaligned body.

Diagram 2 shows ideal alignment. To begin, check yourself sideways in a mirror. Imagine a string on the top of your head gently lifting it upwards towards the ceiling. At the same time, another string runs from below the shoulders down through your lower back, legs and feet into the ground. Or you could imagine pulling a zipper in and up from your bottom hand to the top.

DIFFERENT POSTURES

All of us are born with a particular genetic bone structure, which may not be ideal. We can, however, maximize our musculo-skeletal potential with understanding, training and application.

When you undress tonight, take a look in the mirror as you stand facing it.

Ask yourself a few questions:

1. Is your head tilted to one side?

2. Are your ears at the same level?

3. Is your chin in line with the dip at the top of your chest where your neck joins your sternum (breast bone)?

4. Are your hands at the same level?

5. Are your hands level when you place your index fingers on your pelvis?

6. Do your knees turn in or out?

7. Does one of your feet roll inwards or outwards more than the other?

If you answer yes to one or more of these questions, you are noticing signs of misalignment.

Now turn sideways.

1. Is your chin poking forwards?

2. Do your shoulders roll forwards?

3. Does your upper chest cave in and your mid upper back round?

4. Does your lower back have an excessive arch or look too flat?

5. Do your knees hyperextend (bow out backwards)?

Now take a look at the diagrams on the next page and see which one looks most like you.

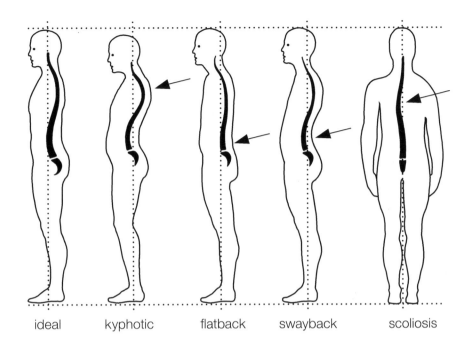

| ideal | kyphotic | flatback | swayback | scoliosis |

When the spine is in its optimal position, you will notice it is not a straight line. It has three curves: one in the neck (a forward curve); one in the mid-back (a backward curve); and one in the lower back (another forward curve).

The curved column of your spine allows your body to absorb stresses and move more freely. However, if you change one of these curves, or if they are exaggerated through poor habits or overused muscles and stiff joints, you will unbalance the whole system.

SECTION 3

Correct and Incorrect Postures and Habits

Our sedentary western culture, with its heavy use of computers, cellphones and other hand-held devices, demands fine-motor and upper-body skills. The importance of the lower body has been lost. We need to re-engage and re-balance the human frame.

You will notice that most of the diagrams in this section are rigid. We have used a puppet to illustrate, first, the compromised positions we often adopt, and second, the ideals we aim for.

When you begin practising, you may notice a rigidity and tension in your body.

From time to time, whatever you happen to be doing, freeze your position. Notice how your body is placed. **PAUSE.** Be aware and make a conscious decision to move towards the ideal. Do this as often as possible thoughout the day and - please try not to be perfect. Just keep practising and soon you will begin to notice the changes.

USING A MIRROR

The use of a mirror is encouraged to give you important visual feedback. Old habits will give you unreliable information, because your brain is used to telling you that the old and incorrect way is the right way.

With regular practice and visual feedback your brain will develop new neural pathways and the new way will begin to feel "right" and the old way to feel "wrong".

By being aware of their own postural shortcomings and making corrections, many of my patients have been able to ease or eradicate their aches and pains.

SLEEPING

A poor mattress or sleep position can give rise to discomfort, which may well last all day.

After waking, notice if you have pain that corresponds to the "ouch" areas on the diagram below.

When you are in bed, see if you are twisting your neck or back or have a lack of support in the area of discomfort.

You may be used to your position and see nothing wrong with it. Study the lines of your neck and back and notice whether they are kinked or unsupported. The aim is to waken in the morning comfortable and refreshed.

Take notice of the front sleeper below whose lower back is excessively arched and whose neck is strained as it rotates to one side in order to breathe.

The position is not restful or recuperative because it compresses certain joints too much.

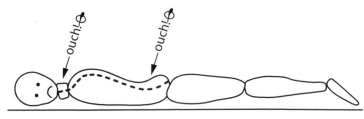

Front sleeper

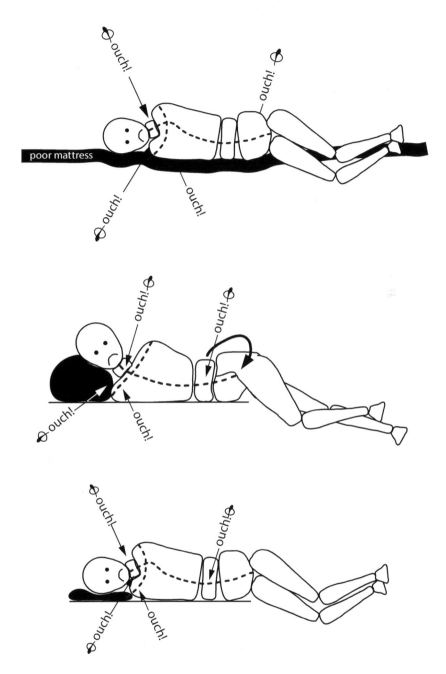

*** continued on next page

SLEEPING - continued

CORRECT

Pause.

A good sleeping position should keep your spine and joints correctly aligned as in the diagrams on the next page. This will help you rest comfortably and allow your musculoskeletal system to restore itself overnight.

Simply changing your old mattress can make a big difference as to how you feel in the morning.

When lying on your side, take the hand that rests closest to the bed and place it under your neck. Feel for any upward or downward tilt on the pillow. There should be no space or lack of support from the pillow at this junction. A good position allows your neck to lie in a straight line from the rest of your spine. The shoulder resting on the bed should not be pulled up towards your ear. If it is, slide it slightly downwards. You may need two pillows above your shoulder or one thicker one for proper support. A rolled-up towel under the top pillow can be helpful to support your neck. Let your cheek rest on the pillow, facing straight ahead. Your neck and back should feel at ease in the morning if you have followed these instructions.

Plumping the pillow or using your underneath arm to support your head and neck are not desirable. A plumped-up pillow will flatten out during the night and you will lose the support. Also, by placing your arm underneath the pillow, stress is put on your shoulder and elbow joint. In this case, it is better to use a second pillow for support.

Some people snore when they sleep on their backs. An anti-snore pillow might help.

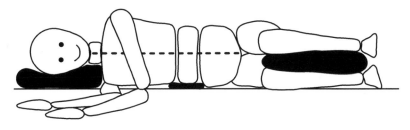

Lie with both knees bent and a pillow between them. You can place a pillow in front of you, so your top arm can rest on it and also prevent you from twisting your torso. Women particularly might need a small pillow at the waist if they feel uncomfortable there.

seen from above

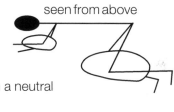

a pillow or two under the head to maintain a neutral head position.

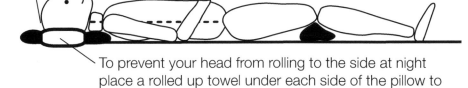

To prevent your head from rolling to the side at night place a rolled up towel under each side of the pillow to form a trough for the neck.

Support options:
A rolled towel inside the pillow case to place under your neck.
Tie a soft pillow in the middle to form a butterfly shape on which to cradle your neck.

★ Each body is different. Use the amount of pillows you may need to keep you aligned, supported and comfortable.

SITTING

INCORRECT

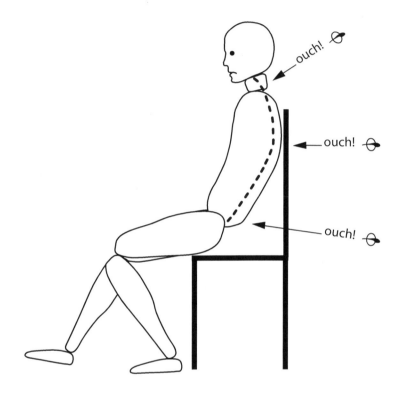

Do not sit on soft deep sofas or low slippery ones. The small of your back will slump and lose contact with the back of the chair. For your spine to be supported, it should be vertical as in the diagrams on pages 40-41. Even if your back is in contact with the chair, it is still possible to sit in a slumped position.

Make sure you are not leaning to one side, i.e. putting more weight on one arm rest. This habit is often responsible for pain in the lower back on that side.

Stand up and move around every twenty minutes!

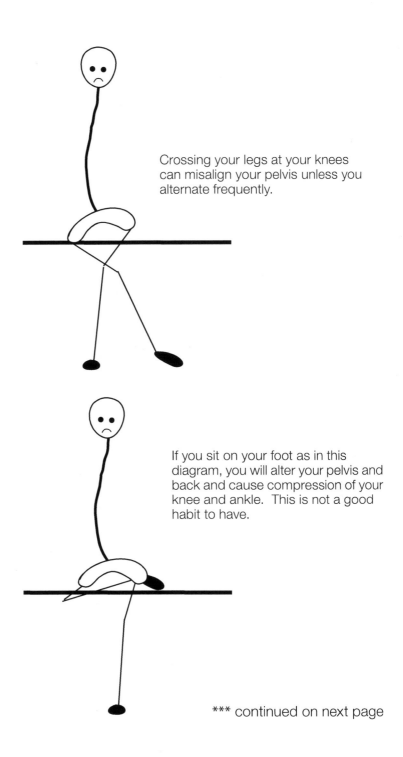

Crossing your legs at your knees
can misalign your pelvis unless you
alternate frequently.

If you sit on your foot as in this
diagram, you will alter your pelvis and
back and cause compression of your
knee and ankle. This is not a good
habit to have.

*** continued on next page

SITTING - continued

CORRECT

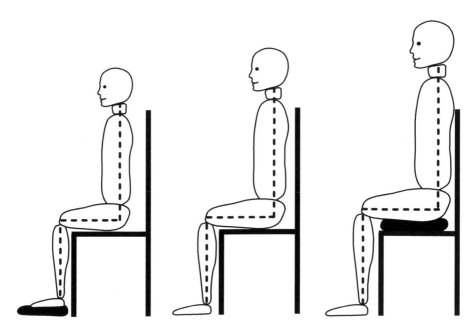

Pause.

Do not sit for long periods. If you must, change position frequently. Get up to move around every twenty minutes or so. If you are short, place a foot rest under your feet. Remember it is there and do not trip over it. If you are tall, you can sit on a firm cushion. People who suffer from lower back pain could place a rolled-up towel or small cushion/pillow in the small of the back for support. Review the neutral spine on pages 38-41.

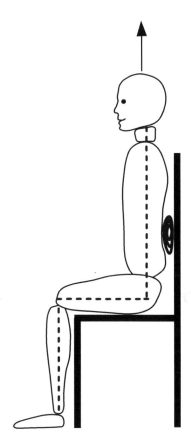

Make sure you sit to the back of the chair and find the neutral spine position (review the neutral spine, pages 40-41). Imagine a string coming from the back of your neck, upwards through the crown of your head to the sky. At the same time allow the rest of your spine to drop towards your tailbone, through the seat to the floor.

Breathe easily from your belly.

 Remember, if you suffer from lower back pain, place a small rolled towel or small pillow/cushion in the small of your back for support.

SITTING AND STANDING

SITTING DOWN

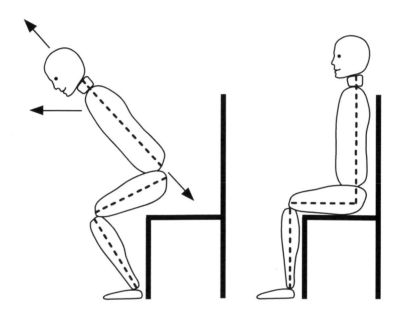

Pause.

Before you sit down, feel for the back of the chair behind your knees for **safety**. Make sure you are balanced and aware of your feet aligned under your hips. Bend your hips and knees slowly so that your body remains balanced. Let your buttocks lead the way to the back of the chair. Feel your leg muscles do the work as you ease yourself **slowly** down. Try not to round or arch your back or tilt your neck backwards as you sit. To remain strong your leg muscles need to work every time you sit or stand. Work on slow, smooth and controlled sitting.

If you fall back sharply into a chair, your head and lower back will over-arch, causing wear and tear on the spine over time.

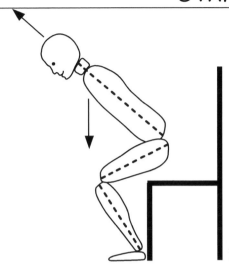

Do not allow your knees to come together as you sit or stand. Instead, keep your knees lined up over the 2nd toe on each foot (see diagram on pages 101 and 151). If you feel shaky or unstable, you can use your hands on the armrests for light support. If you rely too much on your arm muscles to help you, your leg muscles will weaken. It could help to imagine that you are **growing upwards** through your legs as you straighten.

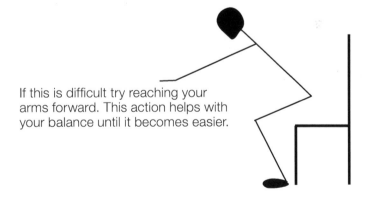

If this is difficult try reaching your arms forward. This action helps with your balance until it becomes easier.

 When you sit or stand avoid using your hands unless your balance is shaky. Bending at your hips and knees will ensure that you keep your legs strong.

WALKING

CORRECT

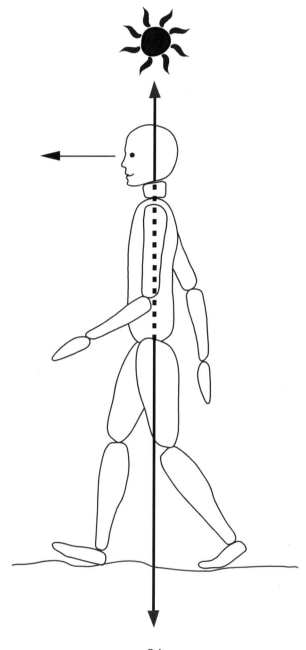

It is important to be aware of our surroundings when we walk.

Take the opportunity to stimulate your senses.
Look with soft eyes
Listen to everything
Smell everything
Feel the ground beneath your feet.

Most of our balance mechanism relies on visual cues to keep us upright. Also, our inner ears are constantly registering our body's position. The inner ears are designed to function best with the head, neck and spine vertical. If we look with our head forward and down, or pulled back, looking up, the sensors in our inner ears are no longer in an optimal position.

To ensure that your walking is efficient and enjoyable, maintain your body in a balanced and relaxed way.

As you step forward let the outer edge of your heel softly touch the ground first, then let your foot roll to the inner edge of the sole and then to the big toe. This rolling action (pronation) allows for shock absorption and good balance.

Jamming your heels down is hard on your body. Try to feel a lightness in your joints.

When walking fast, take quicker steps and shorten your stride. This pace prevents jarred ankles, knees and shins.

Power comes from pushing off with your back leg and foot rather than pulling from the front.

Review pages 38-45 for posture, pages 146-147 for stretching the achilles tendon, pages 152-153 for balance exercises.

★ Be aware of your surroundings as you walk.

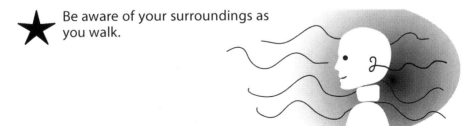

65

WALKING UP STAIRS

INCORRECT

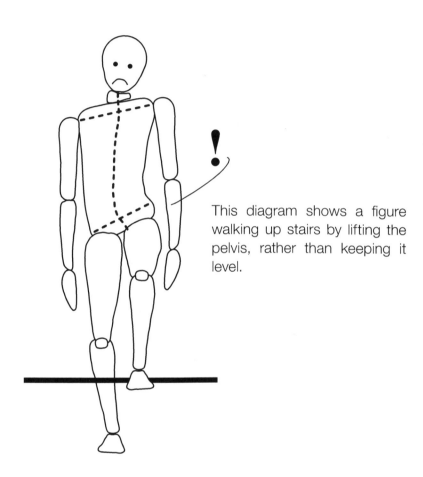

This diagram shows a figure walking up stairs by lifting the pelvis, rather than keeping it level.

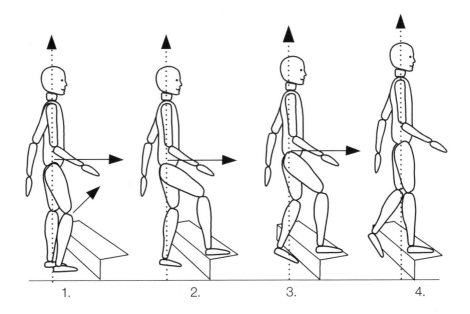

Pause.

1. First bend your front knee

2. Raise your foot onto the step, by lifting your thigh while keeping your torso vertical

3. Carry your body forward towards the front knee, at the same time pushing off from the back foot

4. Now straighten the front thigh. Firm your belly while your back knee and hip come forward onto the next step.

 It can help to imagine you are carrying a tray full of glasses in front, taking care, and keeping it level.

DRIVING A CAR

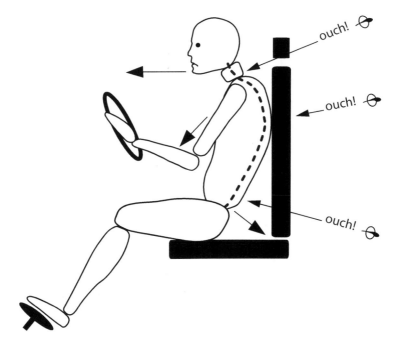

If you slump, your lower back is not supported by the car seat. You may feel pain or stiffness during or after your ride. If you sit in this position and feel no pain you are still contributing to some wear and tear that will become apparent later on.

Notice in the diagram above the mid back rounding and the chest aiming towards the thighs.

The chin is poking forward here, so that the muscles at the back of the neck are shortening and compressing joints and discs.

Also, over gripping the steering wheel transmits tension up to your neck and shoulders.

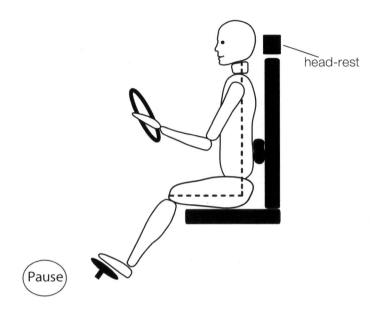

head-rest

Pause

Sit with your hips, spine, neck and head aligned and relaxed (review the neutral spine on pages 40-41). Place a rolled-up towel or small pillow/cushion in the small of your back if you have pain, or will be driving a long way.

Your head-rest should be level with your ears when your neck is lengthened upwards. The level of the head-rest is important. It can minimize whiplash in case of an accident. Be careful not to let your chin poke forwards! Relax your shoulders.

Hold the steering wheel lightly and securely with no added tension to your arms, shoulders or neck.

Drive with soft eyes. In other words, allow your eyes to scan a wider field of vision.

Breathe regularly from your belly and concentrate on the road. Keep your mind uncluttered with thoughts, so you arrive at your destination with a quiet mind and a relaxed body.

TELEPHONING AND TEXTING etc.

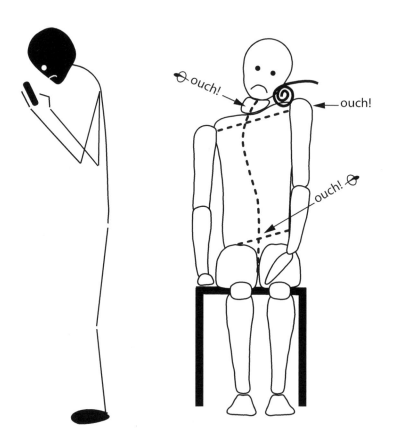

TEXTING: The head is forward from the trunk, the shoulders are elevated and the upper back rounded. This position causes fatigue, stress and strain on the upper body.

TELEPHONING: This diagram shows the head crooked towards the shoulder. This position compresses your joints and discs. The muscles shorten on that side and place an uneven pull on your neck, with the inevitable aches and pains.

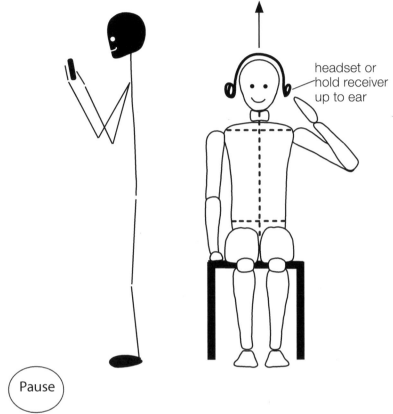

headset or
hold receiver
up to ear

Pause

TEXTING: Bring the device towards you, relax your shoulders back and down and try to keep your head and neck balanced. While using your thumb and fingers to text, try to relax your forearms, elbows and wrists, so you do not over-work. Take frequent breaks.

TELEPHONING: While you are on the phone, keep your neck long and relaxed and bring the phone to your ear. **DO NOT** bring your ear down to the phone. Hold the phone lightly to reduce tension in your arm, shoulder or neck on that side. Avoid crossing your legs.

Be especially careful on a cell phone.

★ Use a headset or earbuds/earphones if you are on the phone a lot.

COMPUTER WORK - desktop

INCORRECT

The chin in this diagram is poking forwards and the middle and lower back is rounding. This position stresses the joints where the **ouches** are.

If the mouse arm is always stretched forwards and away from the body, it causes overuse of the shoulder and makes you prone to neck, shoulder, elbow and wrist problems.

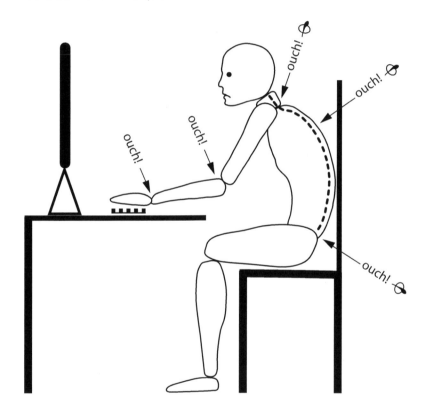

A Sit/stand simple furniture option (see page 171 resources)

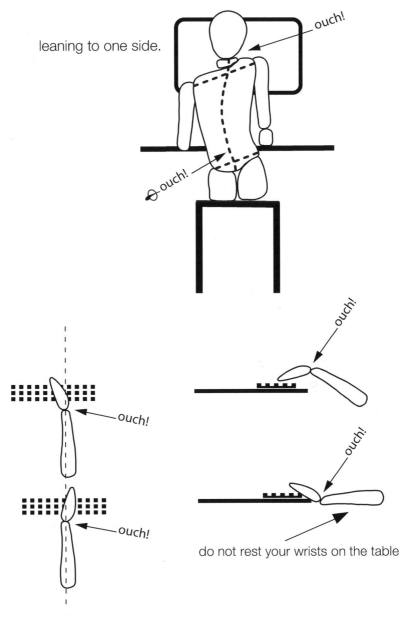

leaning to one side.

ouch!

ouch!

ouch!

ouch!

ouch!

ouch!

ouch!

do not rest your wrists on the table

*** continued on next page

CORRECT

For your spine to be aligned correctly while sitting at the computer, make sure the **back** of your neck is long (review page 142) but relaxed. Maintain your spine in a vertical position, as in the diagrams on the opposite page. Relax your shoulders and be aware of keeping your pelvis level.

Invest in a comfortable, supportive chair. Sit to the rear of your chair while pulling it close to your work surface. If you are experiencing lower back pain, place a rolled-up towel or small pillow/cushion in the small of your back. Review the neutral spine diagram on pages 40-41.

Your elbows should lie at 90-100 degrees to the table and your work surface should be clear enough to allow you to slide your forearms freely left and right in front of you. Your hands should be in alignment with your forearms - not bending upwards or downwards. Poor postioning of the wrists can promote carpel tunnel syndrome over time.

Take frequent breaks while at your computer - ideally every 20-30 minutes. It is crucial to maintain your body's optimum position within the furniture without unnecessary tension. Even if you buy the best ergonomic furniture, it is still possible to sit poorly.

Do not cross your legs or sit on one leg - **EVER!** Crossing your legs alters the alignment of your pelvis and spine. Sitting on your lower leg compresses the knee joint, which produces stress on both your knee and back. It also compromises circulation.

Wheels on the computer chair are there to assist you to move easily if you are doing various tasks from side to side or forwards and backwards.

Make sure you use your feet, knees and hips to move the chair, but maintain your spine in an upright position without twisting when moving side to side or forwards and backwards.

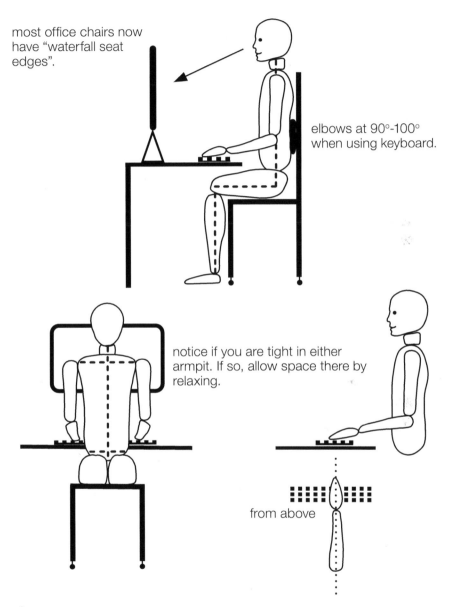

most office chairs now have "waterfall seat edges".

elbows at 90°-100° when using keyboard.

notice if you are tight in either armpit. If so, allow space there by relaxing.

from above

★ Maintain the optimal position for your body within the furniture. No drooping or lolling to one side.

Get up and move frequently.

COMPUTER WORK - laptop

INCORRECT

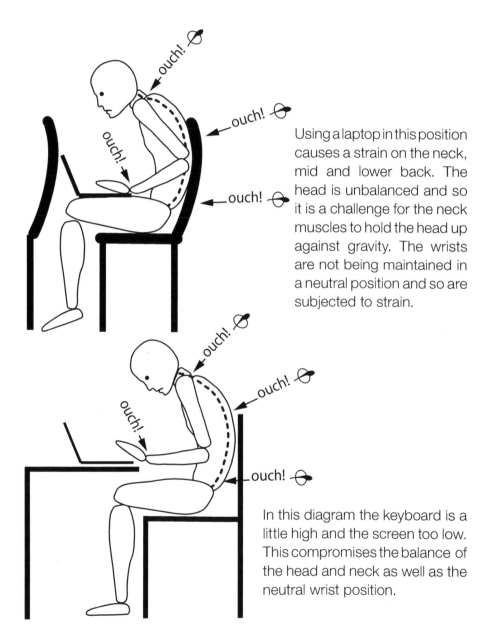

Using a laptop in this position causes a strain on the neck, mid and lower back. The head is unbalanced and so it is a challenge for the neck muscles to hold the head up against gravity. The wrists are not being maintained in a neutral position and so are subjected to strain.

In this diagram the keyboard is a little high and the screen too low. This compromises the balance of the head and neck as well as the neutral wrist position.

Pause

Three options for laptop use:

1. Place your laptop on a stable surface with reams of paper or a phone book to raise it up. Find a position in which the keyboard is not too high and the screen not too low. Use a mouse on the table top.

2. Use a foot rest to raise the slant of your thighs.

3. Place an empty 2-3 inch ring binder, with the thicker edge towards your knees under the laptop.

In these positions, have your head and neck in balance, shoulders relaxed, spine lengthened and released down into your sit bones and your weight into the feet.

For prolonged periods of laptop use, attach a regular size external keyboard tray, positoned slightly below elbow height. Angle the screen to reduce any forward bend of your head. Look down with your eyes. Use a document holder vertically to assist you in maintaining a neutral neck position.

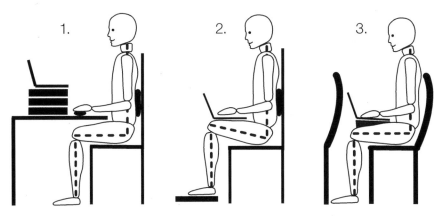

Take frequent breaks every 20 minutes to stretch and move around. Carry your laptop in a wheeled case or a backpack (over both shoulders). Eliminate carrying your laptop whenever possible by using a memory stick, flash cards or a virtual portal.

WRITING
INCORRECT

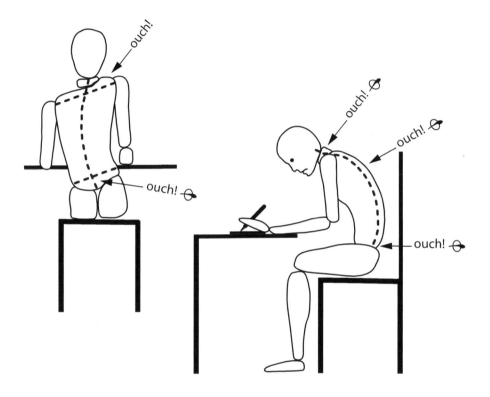

The diagram on the left shows a back view of the body leaning and twisting. We often do this because we tilt the paper, tilt our bodies, and end up with our heads cocked to one side, in order to see what we are writing,

In the side view on the right, the head is forward and down and the spine rounded. The **ouches** show areas of stress.

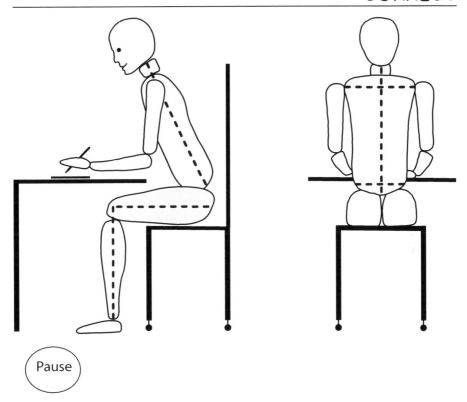

(Pause)

Align your spine, neck and head. Rotate the paper rather than your body. Rock forwards from your hips keeping your spine straight. Look down with your eyes not your head. Relax your shoulders, allow weight to drop into the elbow so that your wrist is freer to move. Hold the pen lightly in your hand and let your writing arm move easily across the paper by opening your shoulder outwards, effortlessly.

If you have some pain in your thumb, fingers or hand, you could buy a pen or pencil grip. Most stationary stores carry them.

Correct angle of paper seen from above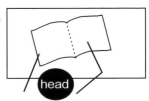

READING, KNITTING etc

INCORRECT

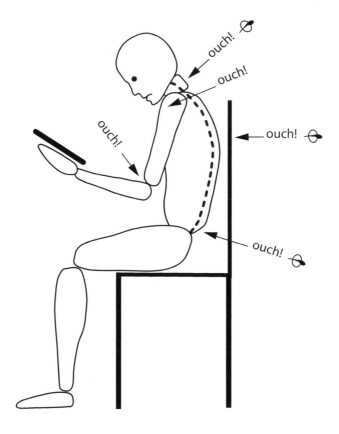

Many people let their heads drop forward and their mid-backs round in order to look down at their book or handiwork. This position leads to overworked muscles.

Also if your lower back is slumped away from the back of the chair, mechanical stress acts on your spine.

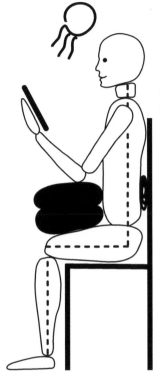

Use a chair with a firm seat and back support. Arm rests can be useful to contain the pillows.

Sit to the rear of the chair with your spine vertical.

If you have lower back pain, use a rolled up towel or pillow/cushion in the small of your back.

While you hold your book or knit, place 1 or 2 pillows on your lap to support your elbows so you can relax your shoulders. Keep your head balanced on your neck (review neutral neck position on page 142) and use your eyes, NOT YOUR HEAD, to look.

You could imagine weight dropping into your sit bones and feet. Keep the front of your chest open. Breathe deeply from your belly and relax without slumping.

 To reduce strain while reading, bring the book up to your head not your head down to the book. Take frequent breaks.

WATCHING TV etc.

INCORRECT

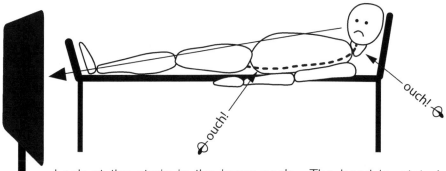

Look at the strain in the lower neck. The head is rotated towards an off centre TV.

This position causes neck pain, headaches, eventual wear and tear and even pinched nerves.

Avoid this position for watching TV, reading in bed or using a laptop.

CORRECT

Pause.

Sit on a firm chair.

Place a rolled-up towel or small pillow/cushion in the small of your back if you have lower back pain.

Do not sit at an angle to the TV - sit straight on.

Get up and move around during commercials. This change of position and movement is beneficial to your joints, muscles and circulation. Do not lean off to one side on one armrest.

Limit your time or avoid sitting on soft sofas.

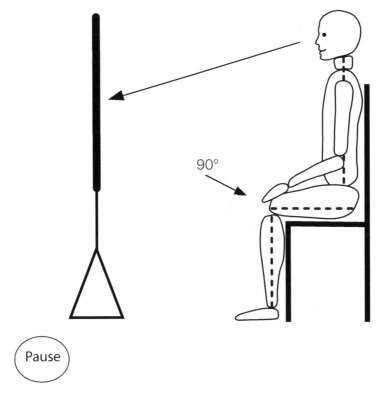

(Pause)

Watching TV from the couch

Position your body so you look directly at the TV. Support your upper body and neck with staggered pillows so that your spine is straight.

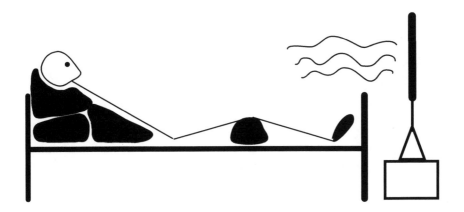

HOMEWORK IN BED

INCORRECT

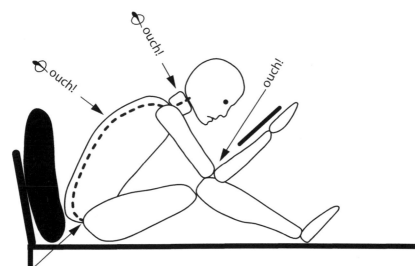

ouch!

ouch!

ouch!

ouch!

Look at the dropped head and the rounded back. This strained position could cause a burning sensation in your mid back. This can lead to headaches as well as the usual aches and pains.

CORRECT

Pause.

Stagger some pillows behind your back all the way up to your neck so that your spine remains straight and not slumped. These pillows help to ensure that your chin does not poke forwards. You should feel supported and comfortable.

Place pillows on your lap to support your forearms.

Use a clipboard for writing. You can tilt this surface without having to round your spine. Use your eyes to look at your work without bending your head forward. Get up to move around frequently, at least every 20 minutes.

Some computer stores sell laptop desk-pillows.

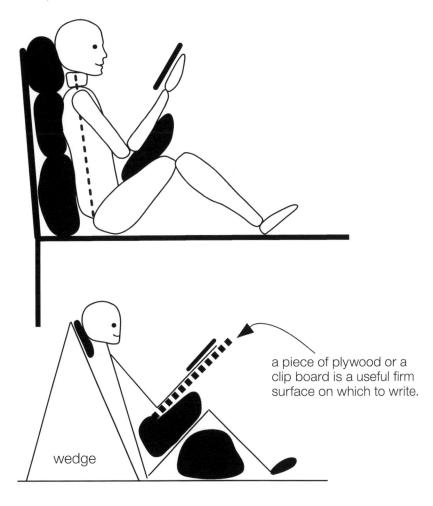

a piece of plywood or a clip board is a useful firm surface on which to write.

wedge

 Use your eyes to look at your work without bending your head forward.

CARRYING A KNAPSACK

INCORRECT

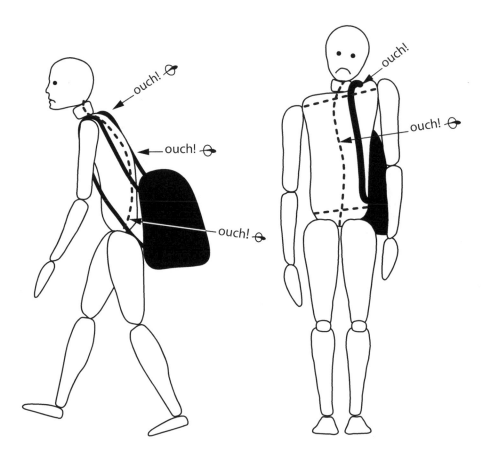

In the diagram on the left the chin is poking forwards and the knapsack is dragging low down on the back. Your muscles have to overwork to counterbalance the weight of the knapsack. You will get a sore neck, mid and lower back.

On the right the knapsack is slung over one shoulder. The shoulder rises to prevent the knapsack from slipping off. The muscles on that side are overworked and the body becomes unbalanced.

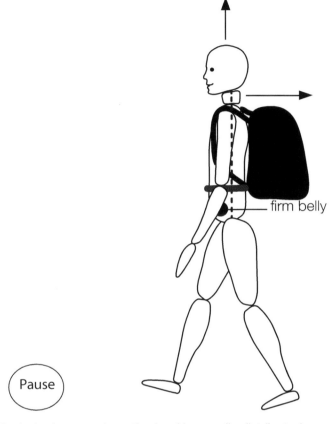

firm belly

Pause

Pack the knapsack so the load is equally distributed across both shoulders. Carry it high on your back, so the load is not pulling down low.

NEVER carry the sack over one shoulder.

Allow the weight of the sack to exert a beneficial force. Do this by adjusting the straps snug enough to allow for a comfortable downward, backward pull. Use the front strap, if you have one, to wrap around your belly. This gives more support. Be careful not to poke your chin out.

If your lower back aches, firm your belly and review the neutral lower back position on pages 40-41.

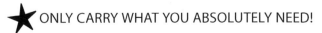 ONLY CARRY WHAT YOU ABSOLUTELY NEED!

CARRYING A PURSE/HANDBAG

INCORRECT

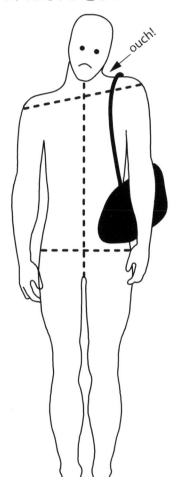

LOOK at the guys on the opposite page. They are holding their purses correctly.

In order to prevent the bag from slipping, many people tighten the shoulder and neck on that side, creating an imbalance. This imbalance can become permanent, causing damage to your neck and shoulder joints.

 Break this incorrect habit and you will decrease much of the strain on your neck and shoulders.

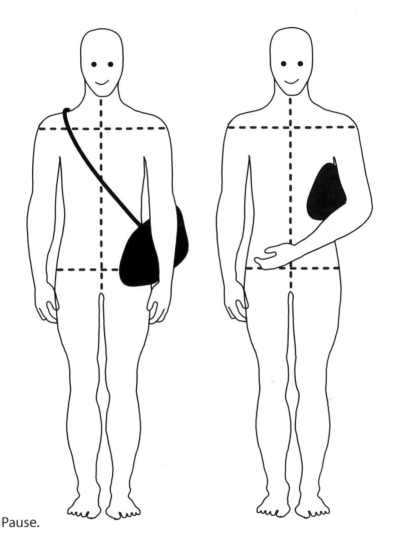

Pause.

Lighten the load by carrying only what you need in your purse.

Either carry the strap across to the opposite shoulder or don't use the strap and **lightly** clutch the purse under one arm.

Remember to relax and drop your shoulders.

CARRYING BAGS

INCORRECT

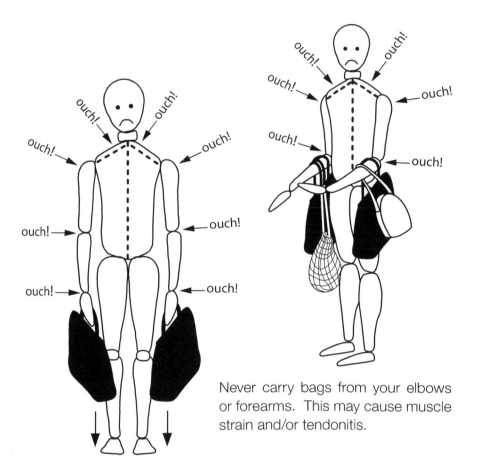

Never carry bags from your elbows or forearms. This may cause muscle strain and/or tendonitis.

The downward pull from the load of these bags puts a direct strain on the muscles in the neck, shoulders and arms and possibly your mid and lower back. Notice the downward angles of the dotted shoulder lines.

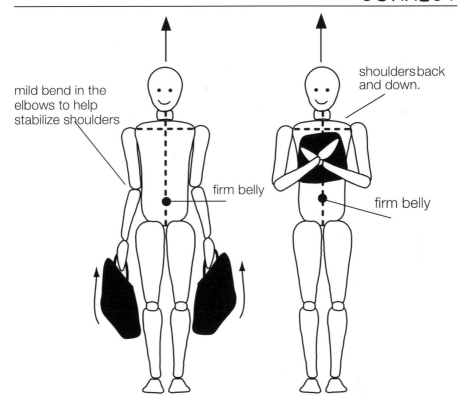

mild bend in the elbows to help stabilize shoulders

shoulders back and down.

firm belly

firm belly

Pause.

Carry 2 bags, one on either side to balance the load.

Have a small bend in your elbows and brace them into your sides. At the same time, brace your shoulder blades together and down and feel the connection of these blades to your upper back (your anchor).

Firm your belly.

If you feel any strain in your biceps (front of your upper arms), put the bags down and rest your arms for a while.

 Stabilize your elbows into the sides of your body while keeping your shoulder blades together and down.

PROLONGED STANDING

waiting for buses, watching sports etc.
INCORRECT

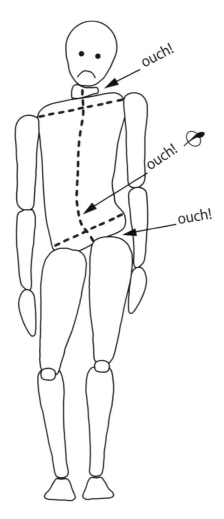

Take a look at the dotted lines across the shoulders, pelvis and hips showing the effects of a shift of body weight onto one leg. There will be some compression on joints in the areas of the **ouches**.

The side view below shows locked knees and an increased lower back curve. This position will create an overload on the spinal joints causing lower back pain. Notice that the belly muscles are not working optimally so the pelvis shifts forward.

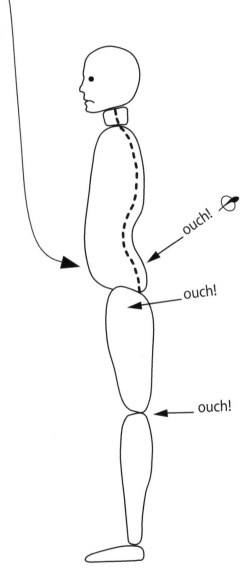

PROLONGED STANDING -
CORRECT

Stand with the neutral spine position (review pages 40-41), with soft knees and an even weight between your legs. If you want, you may shift your weight from one leg to the other as long as you maintain the alignment of your shoulder, hip, knee and the foot.

If you are watching your child's sport and there is an intense moment, relax your neck and shoulders. Keep checking that they are not tensing up.

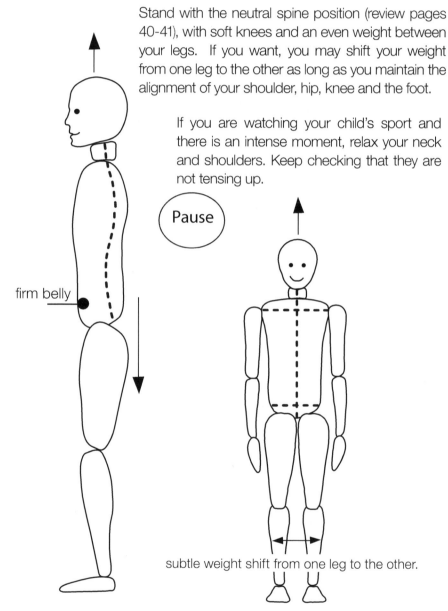

Pause

firm belly

subtle weight shift from one leg to the other.

You could also put one foot, hip distance apart, in front of the other and rock forward and backwards.

If you do shift your weight from side to side, as on the previous page, it might be useful to imagine your shoulders, hips and feet within the boundaries of a picture frame. Do not allow your hips to go beyond the boundaries of this frame when you stand with more weight on one leg. If you have lower back pain, imagine that you are letting your tail bone drop towards the ground. This letting go (review page 143) should reduce the arch and with it the ache in your lower back.

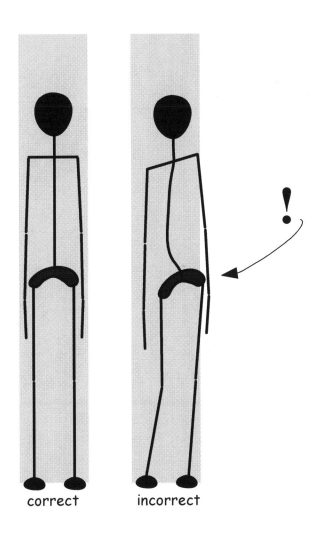

correct   incorrect

STANDING AT A TABLE FOR WORK

INCORRECT

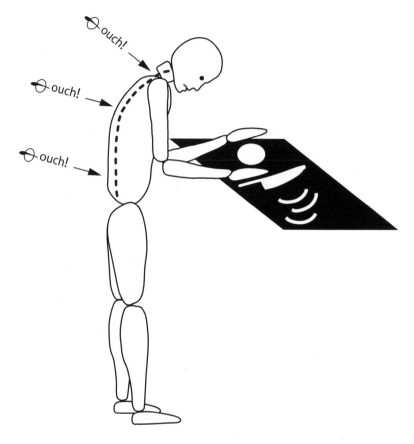

You can see from the diagram that the head is bent forward and the mid back excessively rounded. This shows an unbalanced head-neck-spine relationship.

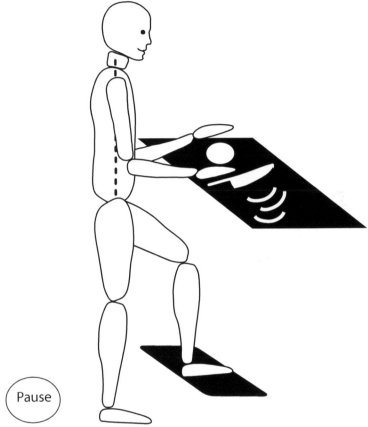

Pause

Keep your head and neck balanced, and your shoulders relaxed. Look down with your eyes and not your head.

Try not to round your mid back.

Firm your belly as you chop.

Place one foot inside the lower shelf of an open cupboard or on a stool.

Stand on a small foam mat if your joints ache after prolonged standing.

Wear shoes with good insoles.

WALKING THE DOG

INCORRECT

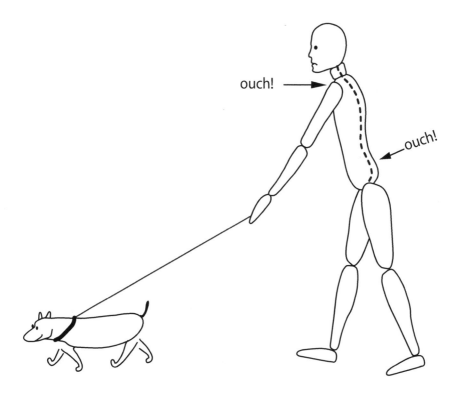

This dog walker has an increased curve in the lower back. The leash arm is forward and away from the body. A sudden yank will increase the arch in the lower back and cause further imbalance. The poor dog walker may get injured, especially with a large dog at the end of the leash.

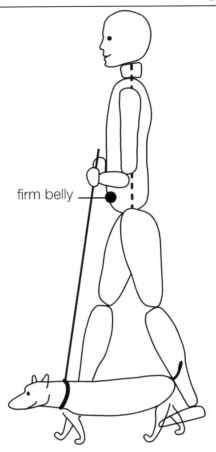

firm belly

Pause.

Relax your shoulders back and down.

Hold the leash between both hands lightly braced against your firmed belly. This method of holding the leash protects your body against an unexpected yank and gives you more control.

Your dog should walk beside you and not be pulling you along. If you need help with this, find a good dog trainer.

Always face unleashed running dogs. Many knee or body injuries have occurred when people are not paying attention and dogs run into them.

LUNGE POSITION

INCORRECT

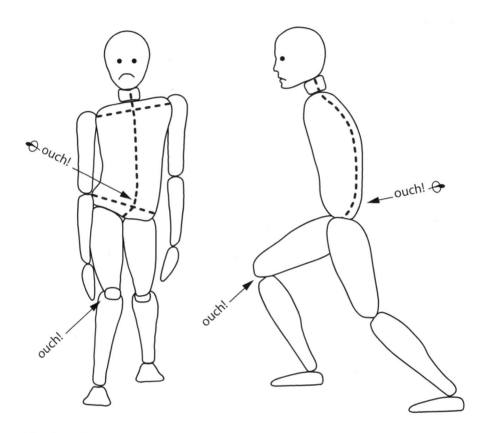

The first diagram shows a front knee dropping inwards from the foot while the pelvis and hip are up and the shoulder down on that same side. This places mechanical stress on the joints.

The front knee on the second diagram is ahead of the foot. This will put strain on the knee. The head is forward and the lower back rounded causing imbalance and poor body mechanics.

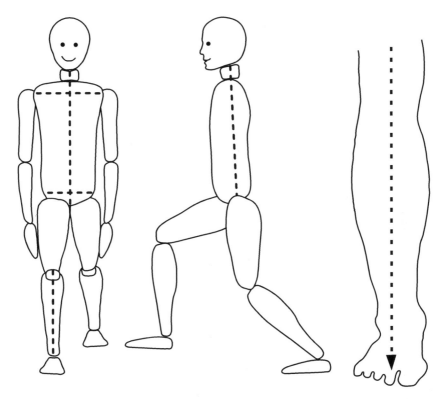

For the lunge position used in some of the diagrams, stand with your feet hip distance apart. To keep your pelvis square, try imagining you have headlights on the front of your pelvis and the beams aim straight ahead. Now step forward with one foot, heel first. The knee should be above the toes and lined over the second toe. You can move your knee back and forth or dip down, but no more than 90 degrees. There should be no pain.

This position is useful for various day to day activities. Try also, to alternate the front knee so that you train both sides. If you feel tight in your calf muscles when you do this then refer to pages 146-147 for calf stretches.

The lunge position strengthens your quadriceps, gluteal and hamstring muscles. Remember to keep your head, neck and spine aligned when adopting the lunge position.

VACUUMING

INCORRECT

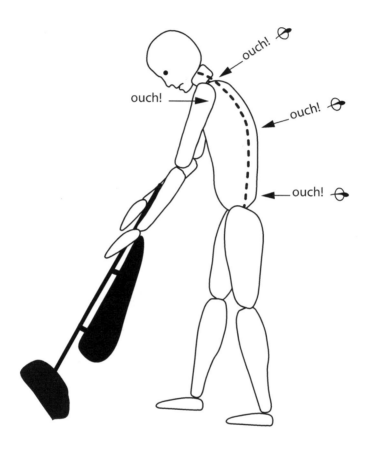

The next time you vacuum, notice whether your head drops forward and your mid and lower back round. If this is so, you are doing most of the action with your upper body and back rather than using your legs. You would be straining your spine and may feel achey and sore.

Pause.

Keep your spine tall and your head balanced comfortably on your neck. Use your eyes to look down, not your head.

Adopt the lunge position making sure your knees are aligned over your second toes (review the lunge position on page 101).

Slide the vacuum forward and back by using a swinging motion of your legs, alternating the bending and straightening of your front and back knees.

Avoid rounding your middle back. Aim your chest, instead, towards the far wall.

Firm your belly. Breathe rhythmically with the movement of your legs.

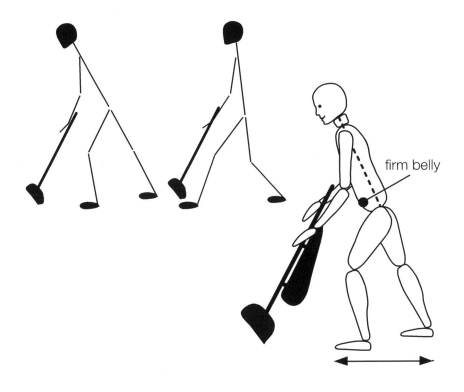

firm belly

PULLING

INCORRECT

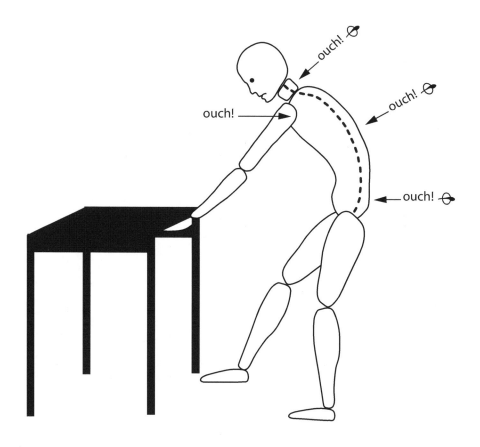

A rounded back with your head looking down will set you up for injury to your spine. Most of the energy is coming from the top half of the body rather than the lower half. Thrusting and pulling actions should come mainly from the legs.

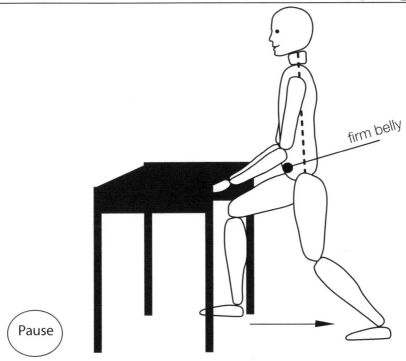

firm belly

Pause

Keep your head and torso in line and your chin tucked in.

Adopt the lunge position (review page 101). Bend your knees as much as you can so that your hands reach the object without rounding your back. Stay comfortably close to the object.

When you are ready to pull, firm your belly while maintaining the neutral spine position (review pages 40-41 and 141).

Transfer the weight to your back leg as you pull. **Try not to round your back.** Pull the load in small movements and check that you are maintaining your alignment and balance.

If your calf muscles feel tight, they need to be stretched. Stretching should be done on a regular basis to be effective. See pages 146-147 for calf stretches.

★ Firm your belly and hold your breath as you pull. This will protect your spine.

PUSHING

INCORRECT

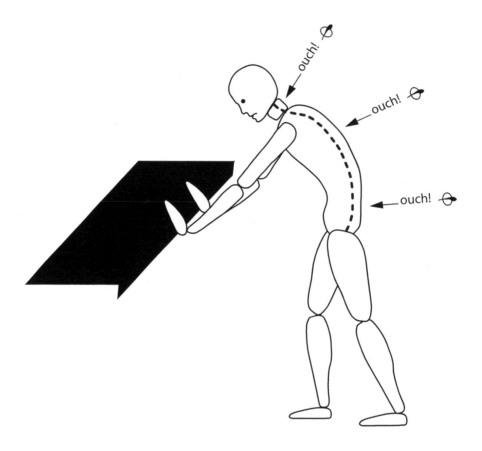

A rounded back with your head looking down will set you up for injury to your spine. Most of the energy is coming from the top half of the body rather than the lower half. Thrusting and pulling actions should come mainly from the legs.

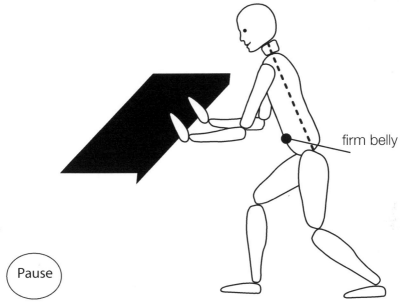

firm belly

Pause

Keep your head and torso in line and your chin tucked in.

Adopt the lunge position (review page 101). Bend your knees as much as you can so that your hands reach the object without rounding your back. Stay comfortably close to the object.

Be aware of your feet rooted to the ground. This awareness can help your balance.

When you are ready to push, firm your belly while maintaining the neutral spine position (review pages 40-41 and 141).

Transfer the weight to your front leg as you push **Try not to round your back**. Push the load in small movements and check that you are maintaining your alignment and balance.

If your calf muscles feel tight, they need to be stretched. Stretching should be done on a regular basis to be effective. See pages 146-147 for calf stretches.

★ The set-ups for pulling and pushing are the same. The direction is opposite.

107

LIFTING

INCORRECT

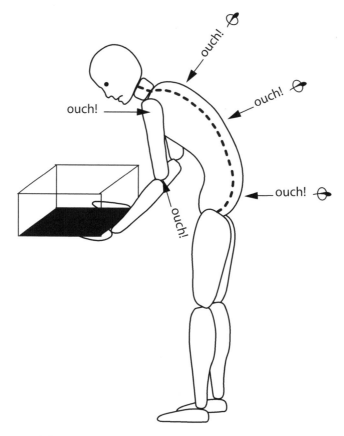

Lifting heavy objects incorrectly causes more damage to your discs than most other activities. It is **very important** to learn to do this correctly.

A rounded back with your head looking down will set you up for injury to your spine. Most of the energy is coming from the top half of the body rather than the lower half.

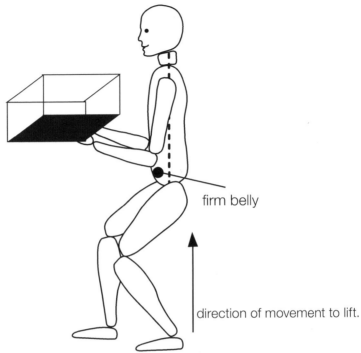

firm belly

direction of movement to lift.

Pause.

Keep your head and torso in line and your chin tucked in.

Move in close to the load.

Adopt a semi-squat position, feet hip distance apart. Bend your knees as much as you can so that your hands reach the object without rounding your back.

As you lift, firm your belly and hold your breath as you slowly straighten your hips and knees, and then breath out. In other words, use your legs to do the work.

 As you begin the lift, if there is any discomfort, lack of control, or if you feel unbalanced on your feet, start again.

PICKING OBJECTS UP OFF THE FLOOR

INCORRECT

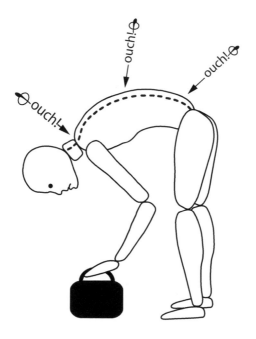

Bending forwards from a rounded spine with straight knees will strain your back. The work is being done from the upper body rather than the strong thigh muscles.

CORRECT

Pause.

Most of us know we should bend our knees to pick things up. But we should also bend from our hips.

Adopt the squat position, keep your spine, neck and head aligned as you slowly bend through your hips, knees and ankles. This will take practise. You can go as low as you are able as long as your back remains straight and your knees stay aligned over the 2nd toes.

Slow down while doing this. Feel the movement in the joints of your legs.

Firm your belly if you are lifting anything heavy off the floor, and keep it close to you.

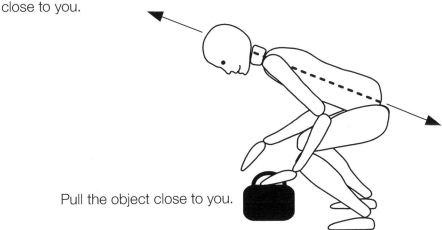

Pull the object close to you.

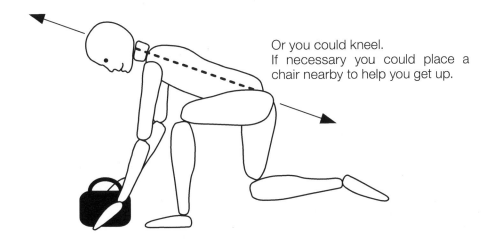

Or you could kneel.
If necessary you could place a chair nearby to help you get up.

 Emphasize the bend from your hips as well as your knees. Your back should remain straight

PUTTING IN OR REMOVING ITEMS FROM A CAR

INCORRECT

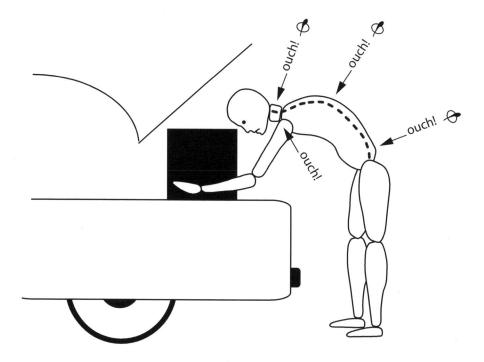

You will be vulnerable to injury if you move items with your spine rounded and your legs straight.

Most people know that they should bend their knees when lifting, etc. But they rarely bend sufficiently from the hips and knees. They continue to round the whole spine too much, with the head poking forward.

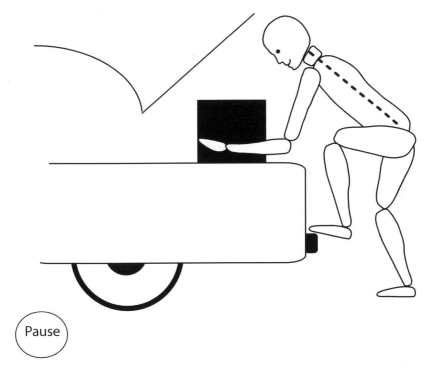

Pause

Place one foot on the bumper if possible.

Slide the items away or towards you, little by little. The further away the item is from you, the more vulnerable you are to injury.

Use your hips and knees to shift the weight.

If you have been on a plane trip or long drive, warm up and walk around a bit before you do this. Your back and hips may be stiff and your muscles tight and this is when injury can occur.

Firm your belly as you shift and do not allow your mid back to become rounded.

BREAST FEEDING BABY

INCORRECT

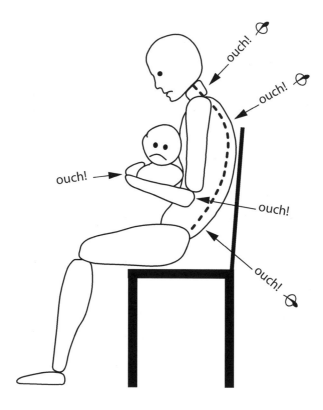

Most women conform their bodies to the baby.

This mother's lower back is unsupported. Her head is dropping forward, her shoulders elevated, her mid back rounded and the wrist holding the baby is overly flexed.

If possible, use a chair with arm rests. Sit back so that you are supported by the chair. Keep your spine vertical (review pages 40-45). Place a small, rolled-up towel or pillow/cushion in the small of your back for support.

Place 1 or 2 pillows or a good nursing pillow on your lap so that the baby is in a position close to your breast. The pillows should help you relax. There should be no feeling of strain anywhere.

Relax your shoulders without slumping forward. When looking down at the baby, use your eyes instead of dropping your head.

Place the baby for feeding where you can relax and be supported well.

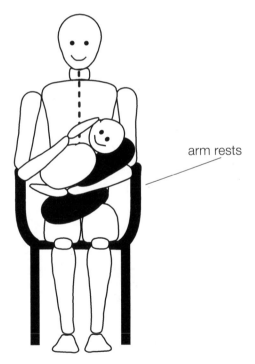

arm rests

 The key here is not to slump your mid back.
You should feel relaxed and supported without strain or tension in any body part.

PUSHING BABY IN A STROLLER OR PUSHING A SHOPPING CART

INCORRECT

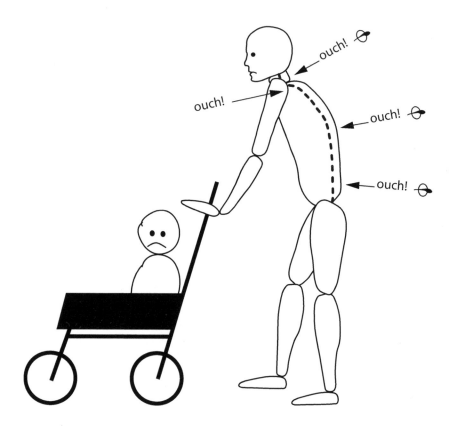

Here, the head is forward, the shoulders are hunched upwards and the mid back is rounded. The person is leaning down into the stroller. Most of the energy and effort is coming through the upper body rather than the lower body.

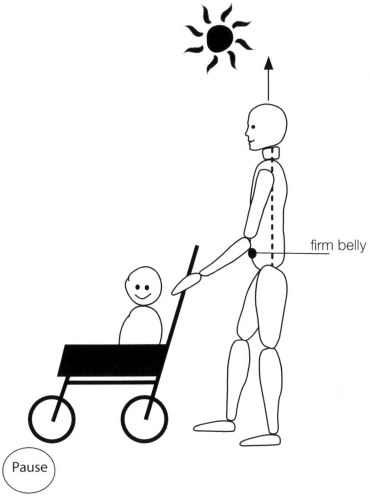

firm belly

Pause

Keep your spine tall and your head balanced freely aligned on your neck.

Firm your belly and push from your legs, hips and knees. Hold the handles lightly and feel a connection from your shoulder blades to your upper back muscles, and from there to your hands.

Maintain relaxation in your neck and shoulders.

CARRYING BABY

INCORRECT

Many women thrust their pelvis forward for the baby to rest on. They also jut one hip out to the side. These positions unfortunately stress the lower back.

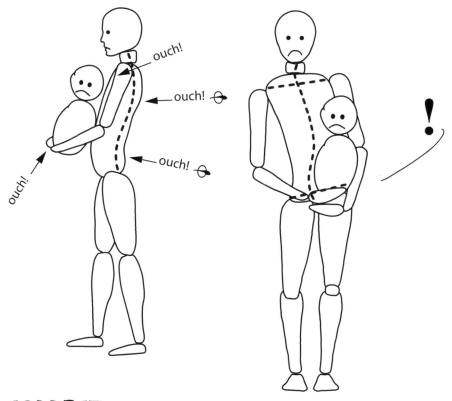

CORRECT

Pause.

Keep your spine tall and your belly as firm as you are able. Review the neutral spine on pages 40-41. Try to protect your lower back by not over arching.

Your body after pregnancy will take time and retraining to regain a balanced center of gravity and core strength. If you are having any problems it is advisable to see a doctor or physiotherapist.

Notice in the diagrams on this page that the shoulders are lined up over the hips. Maintain your alignment as well as you can. Switch sides frequently if you hold the baby on one side. Do not lock your knees.

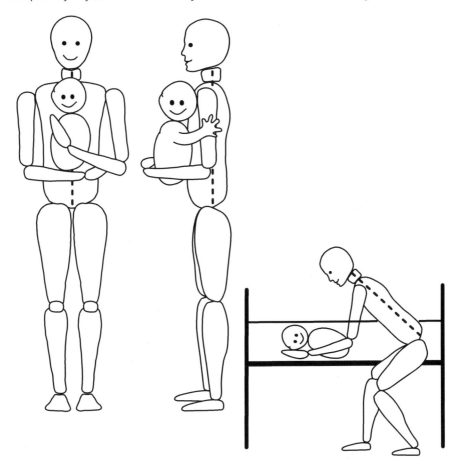

Lifting over the side rails can put excessive strain on your back. Bend your hips and knees when lowering and lifting the baby.

If you carry your baby in a pouch or sling in front of you, try not to let your pelvis be pulled forward and your lower back to arch. If the arch is too great your lower back may hurt. If it does, try firming your belly and reducing the arch.

RIDING A BICYCLE

INCORRECT

Here, the horizontal lines of the shoulders, pelvis and hips are tipped to one side. This position overloads your back on that side. The knee on the downward pushing leg is not centered over the middle of the foot, which may give rise to knee problems.

From the side view, the head is excessively forward and the mid back rounded, which might cause aches and pains in these areas.

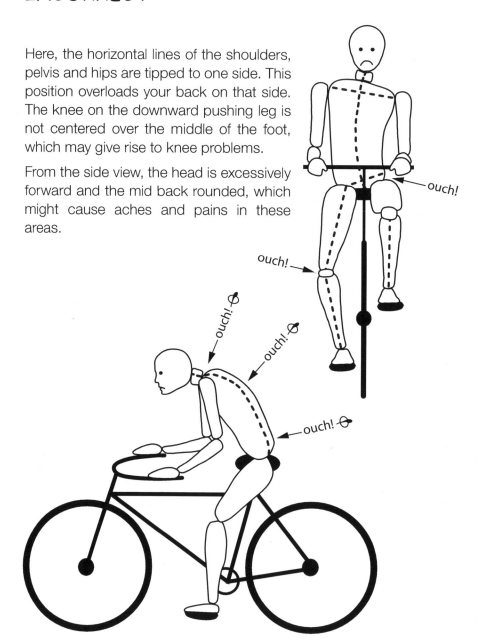

If you are a serious cyclist, you may need a thorough bike/body assessment by a physiotherapist trained in this area.

Your seat height is correct when you have a slight bend in the knee with your foot at the bottom of the pedal's cycle. This will help to maintain a level pelvis. Be conscious of the movement of your hips and knees, making sure your knees come upwards equally on both sides. Align your knees over the second toes while you pedal to protect your knees from strain. Ask a friend to watch from behind to check your alignment.

Try to attain equal weight on your seat and handlebars. If possible, raise or lower the seat/handlebars to achieve this.

Try to keep shoulders relaxed and level and your chin from poking forward.

If you bicycle faster, lean forward through your hips rather than rounding your back and shoulders.

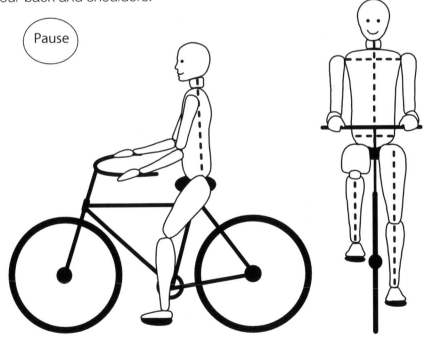

 Feel strong in your core/middle while you push with your legs and hips and keep the upper body relaxed.

SHOVELLING SNOW

INCORRECT

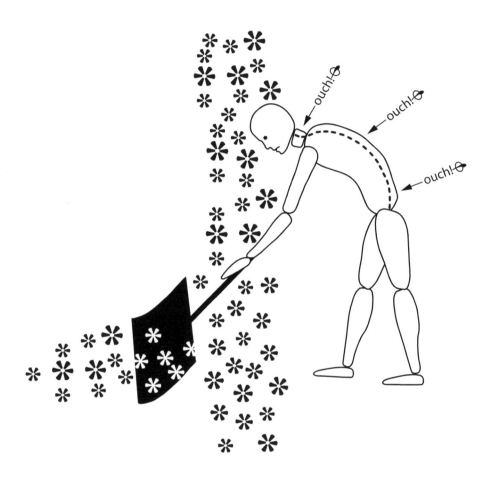

This diagram shows the movement coming from the upper body. When the knees are straight, they are unable to exert a good thrust on the shovel.

When shovelling is done incorrectly, many people end up in the doctor's or physiotherapist's office with injuries.

Warm up first to get your blood circulating and your muscles warm. Try some calf stretches (review pages 146-147) prior to doing this job.

Place your feet in a lunge position with your spine, neck and head aligned.

Keep the shovel comfortably close to your body and firm your belly as you push the snow with your hips and knees. In other words, really make sure you feel your lower body is doing most of the work.

If you are just pushing snow, keep the shovel close to your body and try not to let any part of your back round.

Do this in stages, taking frequent breaks. This is strenuous and taxes your heart, circulation and musculo-skeletal system. Many people are not conditioned for this.

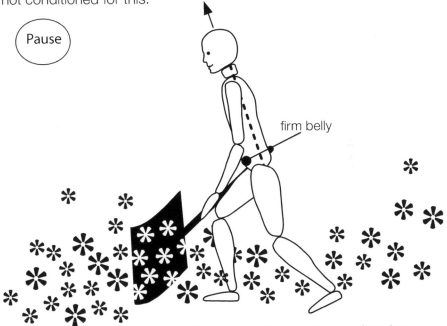

Pause

firm belly

keep the shovel fairly close to your front leg

★ It is not only old people who have heart attacks.

*** continued on next page

CORRECT

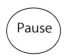

Pause

If you wish to throw the snow straight ahead, bend your knees deeper, maintain a firm belly and straight back. Lift the shovel as you bring it closer. Throw the snow forward when you transfer your weight from the back to the front leg.

If you wish to throw the snow in another direction, turn by **stepping** rather than twisting your body. If you twist, you are likely to injure your back or knees.

To maintain symmetry, change hands and leg position frequently.

Take frequent breaks.

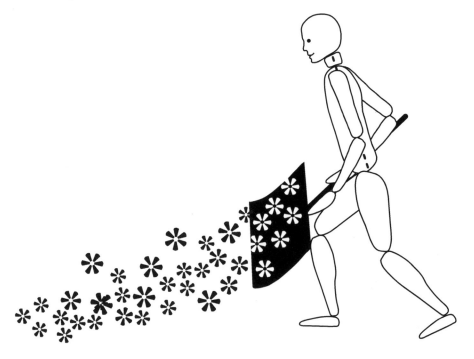

As an alternative position for lifting you could use the squat position

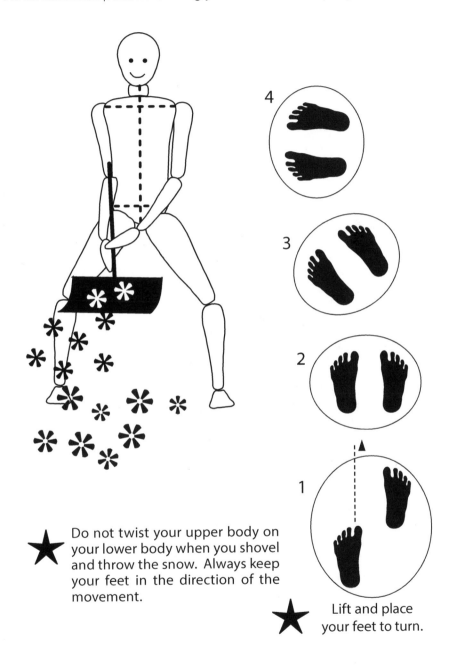

4

3

2

1

Do not twist your upper body on your lower body when you shovel and throw the snow. Always keep your feet in the direction of the movement.

Lift and place your feet to turn.

PUSHING A WHEELBARROW OR LAWN MOWER

INCORRECT

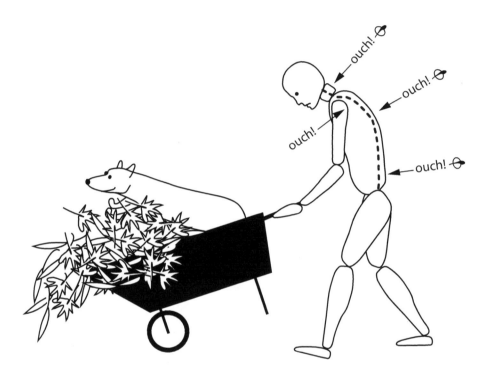

This diagram shows someone looking down by dropping their head and neck and rounding their back. The exertion then comes from the upper body. This strains the neck and back and is very tiring.

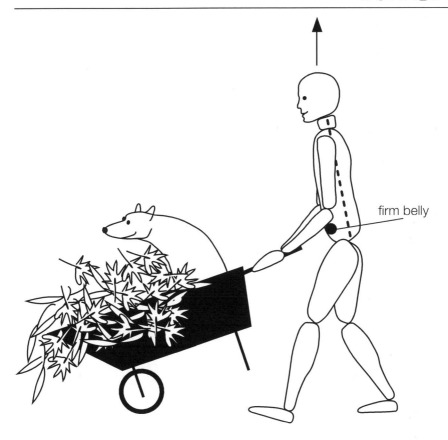

firm belly

Pause

Align your spine, neck and head. Relax your shoulders and be aware of the connection of your shoulder blades to your upper back and down from there to your hands.

Move in close towards the barrow or mower, firming your belly so that you can push with your legs rather than your upper body.

 Balance your body and the load before pushing.

GARDENING, SITTING and STANDING

INCORRECT

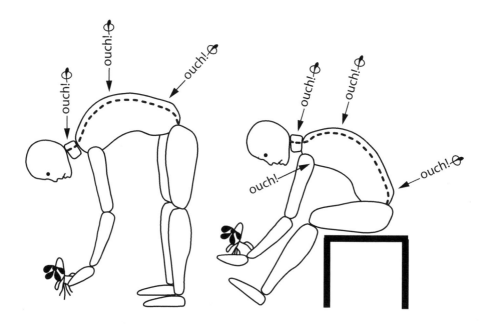

These diagrams show excessive rounding of the spine.

The standing figure is also bending over with straight knees. Unless your hamstring muscles at the back of your thighs are very flexible, all the strain is on your spine.

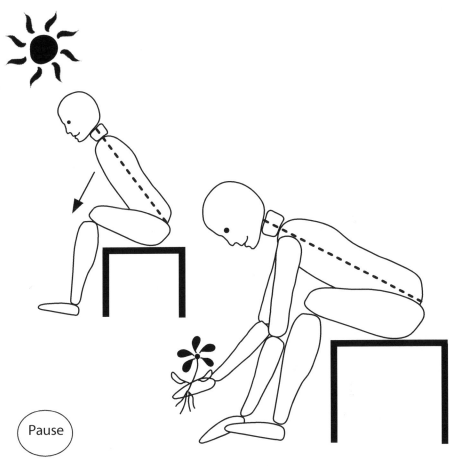

Pause

Gardening should be pleasurable.

Keep your spine, head and neck aligned and bend forward from your hips.

If this is hard for you, work on hip mobility and hamstring and calf flexibility. See pages 146-147 for calf stretches, 148-149 for hamstring exercises and 154-159 for hips.

Take frequent breaks and vary your tasks.

GARDENING, KNEELING and SQUATTING.

INCORRECT

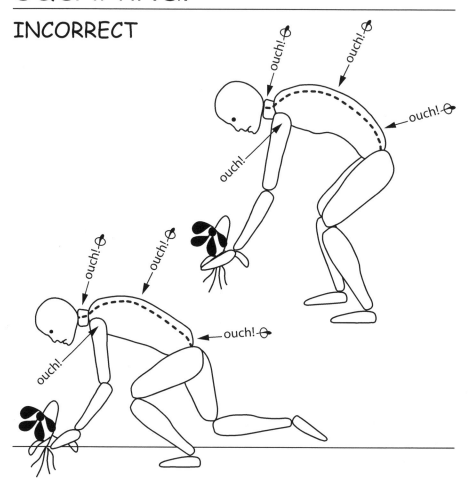

Here the spine is rounded too much with the head poking forward and the body unbalanced. Most of the work comes from the upper body in this awkward position.

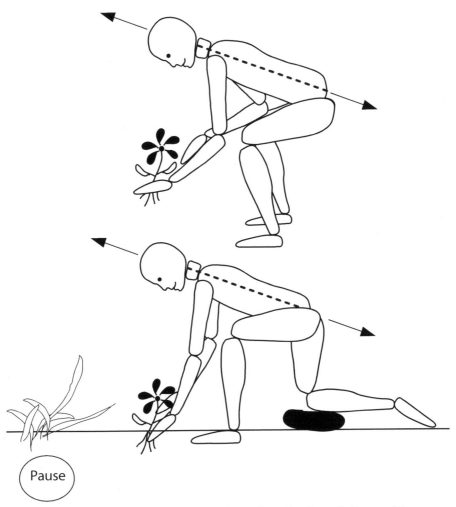

Pause

Keep your back, head and neck aligned and relaxed. If squatting, you may rest one elbow on your thigh. If kneeling, allow your torso and thigh to make contact as you reach forward.

Use a knee pad if your knees are sensitive. Alternate legs.

Move forwards and backwards only. If you have to overreach or move sideways, stand up first and then reposition.

Take frequent breaks and vary your tasks.

GARDENING, DIGGING, SHOVELLING

INCORRECT

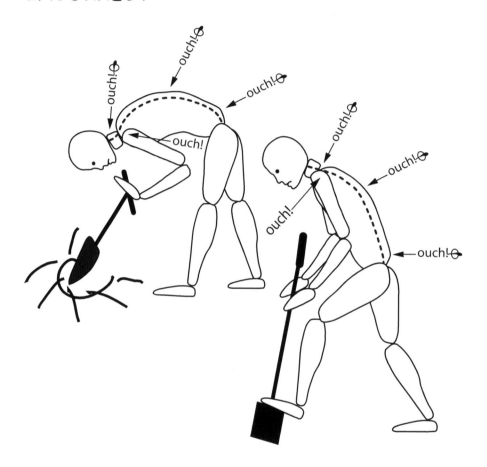

With an excessively rounded spine and straight knees, I will likely be seeing you in my clinic.

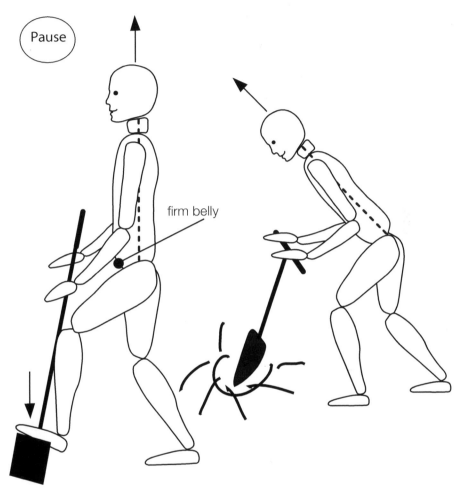

Keep your back, head and neck aligned and relaxed.

Adopt the lunge position (review pages 100-101). Firm your belly and feel the thrust from your hips and knees. Keep your shoulder blades back and down without your mid back rounding. Try to alternate legs, so that both are worked equally.

 Take frequent breaks and perform other tasks in between.

GARDENING, RAKING LEAVES

INCORRECT

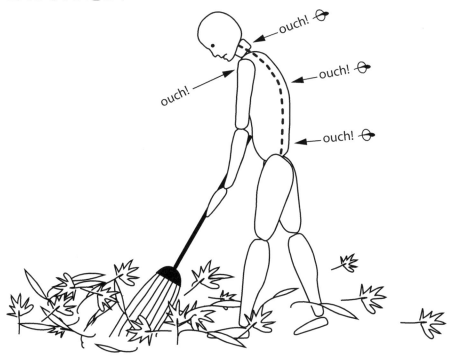

This excessively rounded spine and straight knees will stress your muscles, joints and discs and will cause fatigue. If you twist your spine with your legs straight and your feet planted as you rake, you will further compound the stress.

CORRECT

Pause.

Keep your back, head and neck aligned and relaxed, with your knees slightly bent. You will also be bending slightly forward from your hips. Make sure your spine remains straight.

Now you can shift your weight side to side from one leg to the other. Try alternating your legs so both get equal work. Switch sides with the rake so you use both sides of your body.

You can also step forwards and backwards.

Firm your belly. Relax your shoulders and be aware of the connection of your shoulder blades to your upper back and from there down to your hands as you rake. Tuck your chin in to tilt your head just a little and then use your eyes to look down.

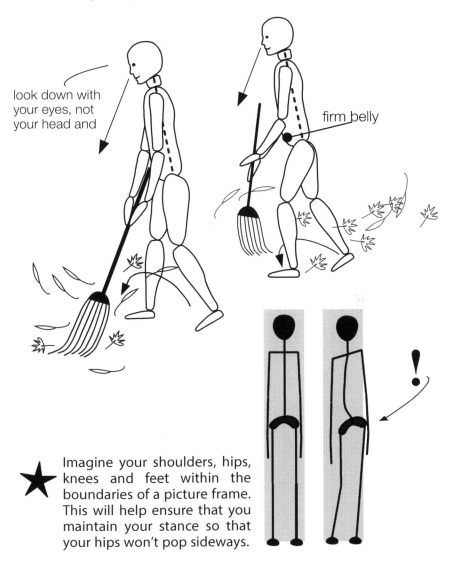

look down with your eyes, not your head and

firm belly

★ Imagine your shoulders, hips, knees and feet within the boundaries of a picture frame. This will help ensure that you maintain your stance so that your hips won't pop sideways.

135

PICKING UP LEAVES

INCORRECT

Bending forward from a rounding spine and straight knees strains your back as most of the work is done from the upper body rather than the strong thigh and hip muscles.

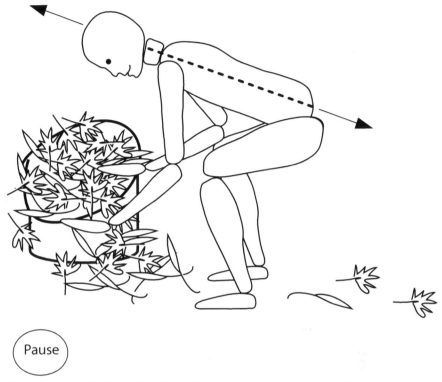

Pause

Keep your back, head and neck aligned and relaxed, allowing your torso and thigh to move closer as you reach forward. You may even rest an elbow on your thigh.

Move forwards and backwards only. If you have to overreach or move sideways stand up first and then reposition.

Take frequent breaks.

SECTION 4

Exercises and Stretching

As we age, muscles take longer to respond to brain signals. Tissues become stiffer and tolerate stress less.

We lose about 30 per cent of our strength between the ages of 50 and 70.

We generally become less active as we age and this contributes to our decreased mobility and power. If we exercise and stay supple and strong we can prevent and slow this decline.

 Often, there are many empty times during the day when exercises can be practised; stopped at traffic light, watching TV, watching the pot boil, etc.

EXERCISES & STRETCHING

For any action we perform (ie. lifting), muscles need to work but not overwork. Our muscles overwork when, while talking on the phone, we scrunch up our shoulder because we are concentrating only on the conversation.

We have 2 approaches to the exercises:

1. Letting go.
   Releasing over-worked muscles (review relaxation on page 31 and muscles on page 34).

2. What we usually consider conventional stretching.
   To lengthen tight muscles.

These are exercises that need no equipment. You can do them throughout your day. They will help keep your body aligned and relaxed.

Correct Method of Stretching:

To make stretching safe, begin with a short warm-up (10-15 minutes), to increase blood flow, tissue temperature and elasticity. A stationary bike, treadmill, rowing, walking, marching on the spot, are ways to warm-up.

Make sure you are clear which muscle you are stretching. Find the correct position for it. Progress will be made easier if you concentrate on the process.

Now move slowly and gently into the stretch until you feel a slight tension in the muscle.

This must not hurt.

Hold this position until the tension passes, then stretch a little more and hold again.

Don't forget to breath.

Do not bounce.

Be patient and consistent with this routine. I suggest using a mirror (review pages 41 and 53).

BELLY FIRMING

Think of your belly as your centre.

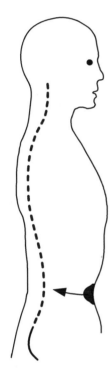

The abdominal muscles support your spine and your internal organs.

The deep abdominal muscle (Transversus Abdominis) is key in postural control and often ignored in exercise programs. This muscle acts like a corset.

Place your hand on your belly and say HAAAH slowly as you breath out. Feel your lower abdomen move in towards your spine. You could pant like a dog using your belly. Or you could think of drawing your belly button in towards your spine rather like the button on a mattress. Hold your belly in for ten seconds as you continue to breathe lightly from the sides and back. Repeat ten times.

If you cannot breathe and hold your belly in at the same time, you are likely working too hard, incorrectly or the muscles are not yet strong enough. Relax and be patient.

Do not tighten or move your back as you do this. If you feel pain in your back, you may be substituting your back muscles for your abdominals.

If you have trouble doing this vertically try lying down with your knees bent.

Do this many times a day, rolling over in bed, sitting to standing, walking, driving, pushing, pulling and lifting. Remember to breathe lightly from your ribs as you maintain this belly firming exercise.

When FIRM YOUR BELLY is mentioned in the book, refer to this exercise.

NECK LENGTHENING

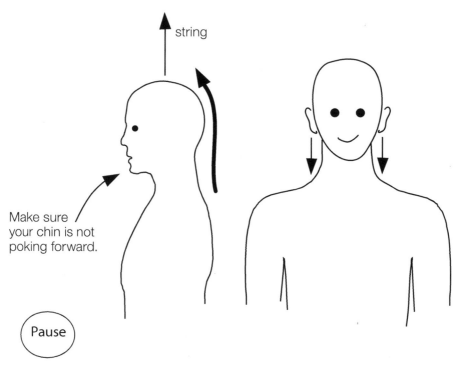

string

Make sure your chin is not poking forward.

Pause

Think of a string attached to the ceiling and connected to the centre of the top of your head. Imagine this string gently pulling your head and the **back of your neck** upwards and slightly forwards without your chin poking out. Allow your face to be vertical to the wall in front of you. Think of "freeing your neck upwards" as you do this.

Soften your jaw muscles by creating a small space between your bottom and top teeth. There should be no tension.

Do this many times a day if possible.

Notice how you react to stress and the effect it has on you, especially your neck and jaw.

 Thoughout the day try to be conscious of any tension in the back of your neck. One sign might be if your chin is poking forward.

142

SPINE LENGTHENING

Pause

Allow the back of your neck to lengthen upwards without tension while the rest of your spine drops away in a downward direction. You could imagine the top of your head reaching towards the clouds, while rooting your lower body to the ground.

Check that your buttocks are relaxed. If you are not sure, squeeze them together, feel the tension, then let them go.

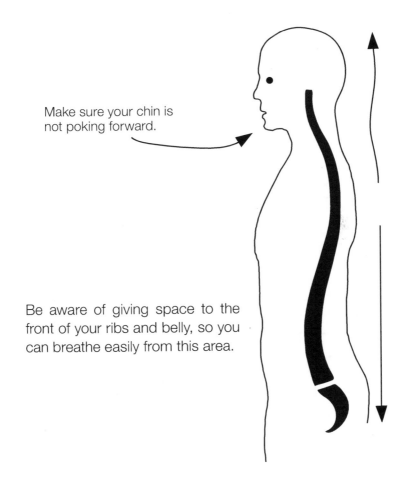

Make sure your chin is not poking forward.

Be aware of giving space to the front of your ribs and belly, so you can breathe easily from this area.

SHOULDER RELEASE

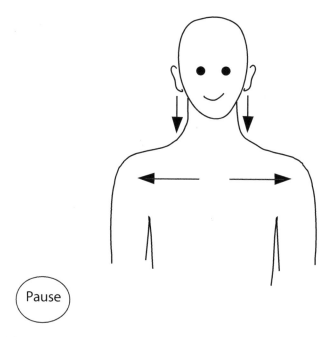

 Pause

Many people have very tight shoulders. In order to counteract this tension, you can do the following exercise:

Shrug your shoulders up towards and slightly behind your ears. Feel the tension in the muscles as you hold this for 5 seconds. Then release them slowly down and outwards.

Imagine that your shoulders are broad and wide like a coat hanger, with your arms hanging loosely down. Maintain a free and lengthened neck while doing this.

Try to do this many times a day and your neck will lengthen over time and you will feel calmer. Keep checking that your shoulders do not creep up towards your ears.

★ Notice what happens to your shoulders when you are stressed.

SHOULDER BLADE POSITIONING EXERCISE

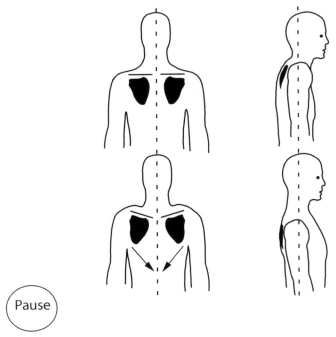

(Pause)

It is important to do the previous two exercises first to set yourself up for shoulder blade positioning.

Maintain the relaxation in your shoulders. With no increased tension, slide your shoulder blades together and down in the direction of your lower back.

Make sure you do not move your spine or upper arm backwards, nor tighten your armpits. Try instead, to focus on the subtle sliding of your shoulder blades. The goal is to feel the connection of your shoulder blades to your upper mid back.

This takes frequent practise. Notice if one shoulder blade slides more easily than the other. If so, try to match them up.

 Remind yourself to do this many times a day.

CALF STRETCHES

Warm up before you stretch (review page 140).

There are two important muscles in the calf, the gastrocnemius and the soleus. They join to form the achilles tendon which connects them to the heel bone.

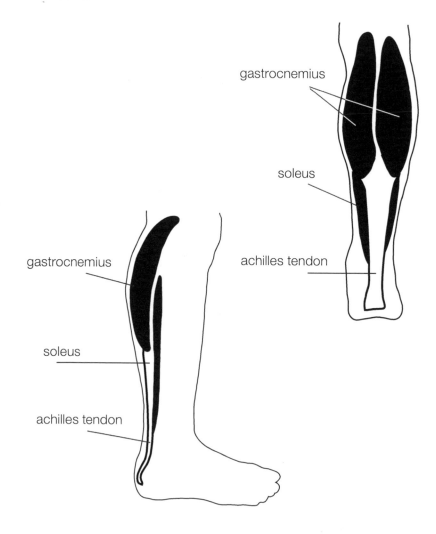

Pause

1. To isolate the **gastrocnemius** muscle you must keep the heel of the back foot on the ground, and the knee **straight**.

Stand facing a wall, feet hip distance apart. Place your hands on the wall.Slide one foot staight back, while keeping your toe and heel perpendicular to the wall and your knee in line with your 2nd toe. Now slowly bend your front knee until you feel a mild stretch in your back calf. Hold for 20-30 seconds and alternate 6 times each side. Make sure your spine, neck and head are aligned, your shoulders relaxed and your belly button is aimed straight ahead.

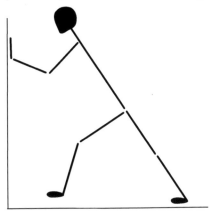

1. gastrocnemius   2. soleus

2. To isolate the **soleus** muscle adopt the same position as above but instead **bend** the back knee 15-20 degrees. Hold for 20-30 seconds and alternate 6 times each side.

Make sure your spine, neck and head are aligned and your shoulders relaxed.

 Do not let your back arch or your hip and back shift sideways while doing this.

HAMSTRING STRETCHES

These large muscles at the back of the thighs originate at the sit bones on your pelvis and insert at the back of the knees. If they are tight they will limit (flexion) of the hips and (extension) of the knees. This tightness will place stress on your back. These muscles also work to control your pelvis and spine.

Preparation.

Pause.

It is important to prepare your lower back before this stretch.

1. Lie on your back with your knees bent, feet flat, hip distance apart.

   Relax your arms at your sides.

   Lengthen the back of your neck, bring your belly button in towards your spine while relaxing your lower and middle back into the mat. Maintain this position throughout the stretch.

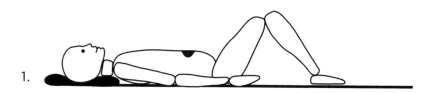

2. Put your hands around your right thigh and gently draw it towards your chest.

   Relax, breathe and slowly straighten out your opposite leg.

   You should feel no pain while doing this, just a mild pulling sensation.

   Hold the position for 10 seconds. Repeat 6 times and then change sides.

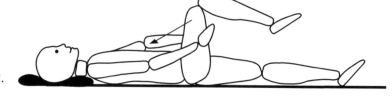

To progress.

3. To target the hamstring muscles, begin with your right leg.

Make sure your shoulders are relaxed on the mat or floor.

Keep your belly button drawn in towards your spine. Maintain the lower back contact with the mat and your neck long at the back.

Bring your right hip up to 90 degrees. Hold the left leg straight down, or as close as you are able, towards the mat.

Place your hands behind the back of your right knee. If this is too difficult, hold a towel around the back of your knee for support. Slowly straighten your right leg towards the ceiling without moving your position. Only stretch until you feel a mild pull in the back of your thigh. Then hold for 10-20 seconds.

Relax and breathe throughout the stretch.

Repeat this stretch 3 times on one side and then change sides.

There should be no pain in your back or your leg as you do this.

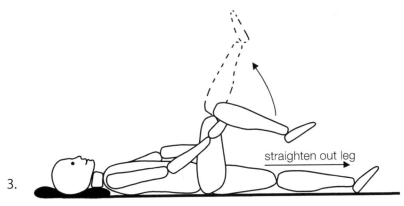

straighten out leg

3.

HALF SQUAT

Strengthens the quadriceps (thigh muscles).

Pause

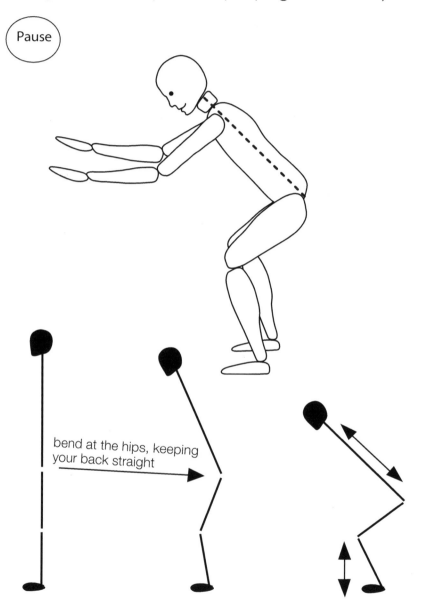

bend at the hips, keeping your back straight

Pause

Ideally, do this exercise without holding on to anything. If you need support, stand behind a stable chair, and hold lightly.

Feel your feet rooted to the ground, hip distance apart. Keep your back straight with your head and neck aligned. Now bend at your hips and knees, as if you are going sit half way to a chair.

Make sure you can feel your ankle joints moving as you bend your hips and knees. Check that your knees are aligned over your second toes, so that the tips of your toes are still visible.

Using your thigh muscles, slowly straighten up until your ankle, knees and shoulders are aligned. Check that your head and neck are in balance and that there is no tension. Do not poke your chin out.

Do this 10 times, gradually building up to 30 or 40 a day. **This should not cause you any pain.** If it does, start with a shallower knee bend and gradually build up your tolerance.

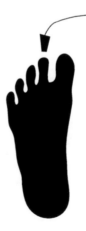

Do this exercise every time you get up and down from a chair and you will keep your leg muscles strong.

BALANCE

BALANCE EXERCISE 1

Stand in a corner with your fingers lightly touching the wall.

Place your feet one in front of the other, heel to toe, and firm your belly while you stand tall, and relaxed.

Look ahead and balance between your two feet. If this is too hard, move your front foot out a little so the feet are not lined up.

Build up until you can balance for 30 seconds and, as you improve, try not to use your fingers on the wall. However, be safe. Do this 3-6 times a day. Change feet.

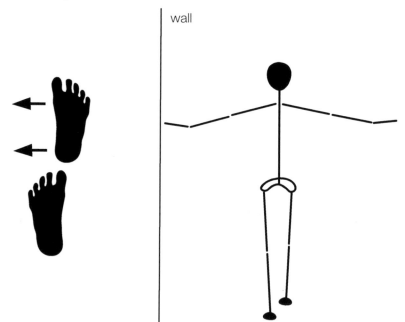

When you feel confident enough, you could progress by doing this exercise with your arms crossed over your chest.

BALANCE EXERCISE 2

Stand on one leg near a wall or in a corner, preferably with bare feet. Do not let your legs touch each other. Look straight ahead and place your fingers lightly on the wall if you need support.

Firm your belly and make sure your belly button aims straight ahead.

The inner ear is an important component of balance. It is necessary therefore, to have your head and neck in the aligned position (review page 44).

Build up until you can balance for 30 seconds and, as you improve, try not to use your fingers on the wall. Do this 3-6 times a day. Alternate between legs and notice if it is more difficult to balance on one side rather than the other. If so, the weaker side will need more work.

Be safe. You could also practise standing on 1 leg when you put your pants or skirt on.

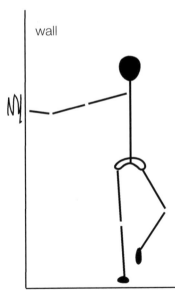

wall

When you feel confident enough, you could progress by doing this exercise with your arms crossed over your chest.

HIP OPENING STRETCHES

 HIP REPLACEMENTS
People with hip replacements must not do these exercises.

The ability to open your hips allows for easier day to day activities, such as tying shoe laces, putting on socks, sports etc.

Remember the "H" line (see page 10)

You may find this exercise difficult. So, I will give you three options:

Exercise 1. The first is for those with very tight hips:

Start by lying on your back, ideally on a firm surface (the floor), if not, your bed. Put a small pillow under your head. Bend you knees at 90 degrees with your feet flat on the floor in line with your hips. (review the H line, page 10). Open one thigh by slowly dropping the knee outwards towards the floor/bed. Place one or two pillows/cushions under that leg to support it, so that it feels comfortable and you are able to relax and gently stretch that tight hip. Hold this position for 30 seconds or so. All the while try not to shift any other part of your body. Make sure not to force anything. Change sides and repeat 6 times on each side. If one hip is tighter than the other, you will need to concentrate on it more.

This will take time and should be pain free. If your hips hurt you should see your doctor or physiotherapist. Later you can reduce the pillow support and then you will be ready for the next option.

You will have to be persistent if you want to progress with this stretch.

Exercise 2.

Start by lying on your back, ideally on a firm surface such as the floor, if not, your bed. Put a small pillow under your head. Bend you knees up at 90 degrees with your feet flat on the floor in line with your hips. Review the "H" line on page 10. Now lift one foot, and place the outside of the ankle on the top of the other knee. Hold this position for 30 seconds or so. Do not move your pelvis, torso or the other leg as you do this. Let your thigh open slowly out towards the floor.

Change sides.

Repeat 6 times on each side, alternating. If one hip is tighter than the other, you will need to concentrate on it more.

You should feel no pain but be aware of the stretch at the back and outside of your hip.

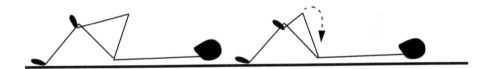

*** continued on next page

continued

 HIP REPLACEMENTS
People with hip replacements must not do these exercises.

Exercise 3.

Pause.

Sit upright in a chair. Keep your back straight and your pelvis level. Review H-line, page 10. Slowly bring the outside of your foot to rest on the top of the opposite knee without allowing your back or pelvis to move. If your hip is tight, you may find this difficult.

If possible, look in a mirror as you do this exercise. It will give you important feedback.

Slowly allow your hip to open. If you do not feel a stretch, bend forward slightly from your hips to bring your torso closer to your foot and knees. Keep your back straight and your buttocks relaxed.

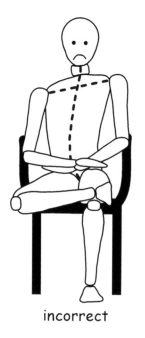
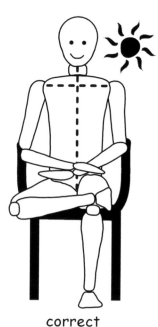

incorrect   correct

Hold this position for 30 seconds or so

You should feel no pain but be aware of the stretch at the back and outside of your hip. Remember to relax and breath when you do this.

Repeat 6 times on each side, alternating.

 You will have to be persistent if you want to progress with this stretch.

Examples:

When tying shoelaces, cutting toe nails etc., remember to bend forward through your hips, keeping your back straight.

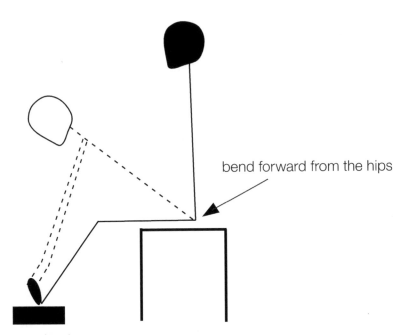

bend forward from the hips

Tying your shoelaces

HIP FLEXOR STRETCH

This exercise will stretch the muscles on the front of your hips. Because we sit so much, these muscles become short and tight.

Do this in front of a mirror if possible and you can place a pillow or mat under your knee for comfort. Warm up first (review page 140).

Pause

Kneel on one knee with your other leg in front of you.

Make sure your belly button is aimed straight ahead and your pelvis square to the wall in front.

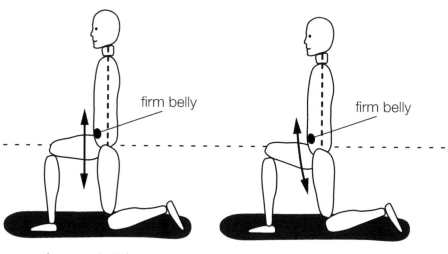

| 1. easy stretch | 2. Medium stretch. |

Keep your belly button drawn in towards your spine, your neck long at the back and your lower back relaxed with no excessive arch.

Slowly sink your hips, so that your weight shifts onto your front foot.

Keep the knee of your front leg aligned over your ankle.

Hold for 10 seconds, while feeling a mild stretch across the front of the hip of your kneeling leg.

Do this 6 times and alternate sides.

There should be no pain in your back or hip while doing this.

Relax and breathe throughout the stretch.

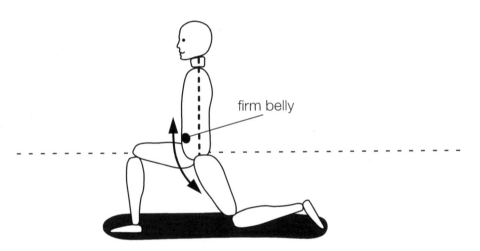

firm belly

3. Advanced stretch.

 Be careful not to arch your back.

OVERUSE OF NECK AND SHOULDERS

Beware of overusing your neck and shoulders on your dominant side in activities such as:

Using your cell phone

Blow-drying your hair

Cooking

Brushing your teeth

Ironing

Lifting a kettle or milk out of the fridge

Pulling laundry out of the washer or drier

Lifting items out of the passenger side of the vehicle (Instead get out and go to the passenger side of the vehicle to remove them).

Notice the head tilting to one side, and the shoulder rising.

Try NOT to do this !

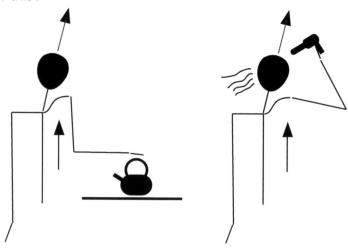

Pause Notice the head is vertical here, and the shoulder is dropped.

Try to do this:

string

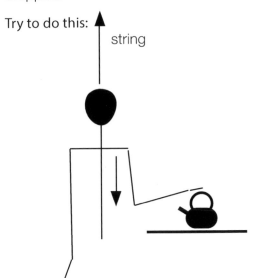

string

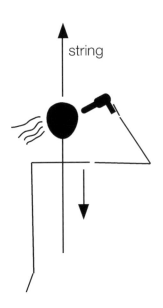

 Think of opening up and moving from your arm pit.

MUSCLE BALANCE

If your body is misaligned, muscle imbalances develop, leading to tension and undue pressure on your joints. For example, a head forward posture causes compensations in the neck and upper back joints.

Common muscle imbalances

weak	tight
neck flexors	neck extensors
rhomboids and lower trapezius	pectorals
abdominals	back muscles
gluteal muscles	hip flexors
quadriceps	hamstrings
dorsiflexors	calf muscles

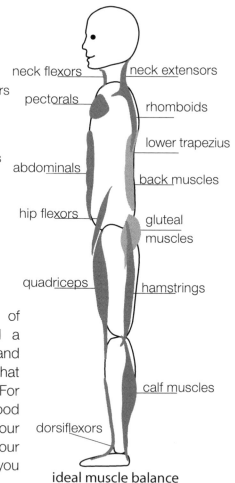

neck flexors — neck extensors
pectorals — rhomboids
— lower trapezius
abdominals — back muscles
hip flexors — gluteal muscles
quadriceps — hamstrings
— calf muscles
dorsiflexors

ideal muscle balance

There are many variations of these muscle imbalances and a physiotherapist can assess and help you to correct yours, so that your body can function better. For the maintenance of your good health it is important to find your centre of gravity and not allow your environment to dictate how you move and place yourself.

CENTRE OF GRAVITY

Your spine should carry your body weight. Looking up and opening your chest can positively affect your mood as well as helping you find your centre of gravity. Imagine balancing and carrying a heavy pot on the top of your head and allowing your spine to carry and balance the load. Or take a wide, open, tall stance and train yourself to feel you present confidence to the outside world!

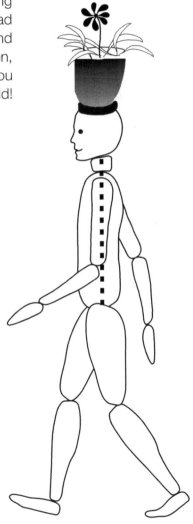

Think of each foot step softly plugging into the ground as you walk. This will help you anchor your base.

PRINCIPLES OF GOOD POSTURE

1. Pause

2. Neck lengthened and released upwards, face vertical, softened eyes, jaw relaxed

3. Shoulders relaxed downwards and outwards

4. Spine lengthened and released downwards into your sit bones and feet

5. Allow space in your abdomen and lower ribcage from the front to the back, to help with breathing, using your diaphragm

6. Be conscious of your movement and aware of any poor positions

7. Be aware of your surroundings and feel confident.

RELEASING TENSION

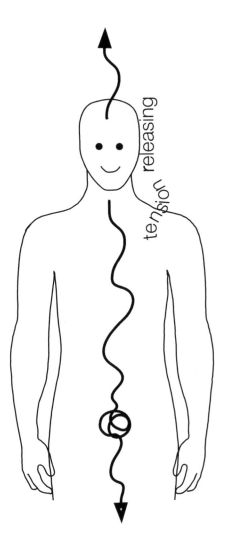

Pause.

Imagine there is a string coming from the back of your neck, lifting through the top of the middle of your head, towards the sky. The string from below the neck drops down through your spine to your tailbone, weighted towards the ground and into your feet.

SECTION 5

Tips, References and Resources

TIPS FOR WALKING WITH A CANE

To ensure that the cane is the correct height for you, stand with your shoes on and your spine, neck and head aligned. Rest the cane against your side, upside down, with your arm hanging over it.

The cane length is correct when the end lines up with the bump on the back of your wrist. If it does not, adjust it and check again.

Make sure you have a good rubber tip on the end and check it regularly for wear. Replace it when needed as it could be the cause of a slip or fall.

The rule of thumb is to place the cane in the opposite hand and side from the one that is painful or weak. But there are exceptions to this. Listen to the advice you have been given.

Do not overgrip with your hand. Relax your shoulders down as you put light pressure through the cane.

The cane should go forward with the opposite leg when you walk. Use it as lightly as is safe. Do not overlean by causing your spine to list. Feel the connection to your shoulder blade while you apply pressure through your hand to the cane. Be aware of your feet on the ground.

Many people put too much weight through the cane, depending on it, rather than working their bodies as much as is safe.

TRAVEL TIPS

When travelling on a long journey by plane, car or bus, in a confined space, it is easy to end up in one position for too long. This will leave you feeling stiff and tired and may even give you muscle cramps. This will be made worse if you sit in a twisted position, lean off centre or fall asleep with your neck and head to one side.

Align your spine, neck and head and place a small pillow or rolled towel in the small of your back. If you are travelling on a plane, a neck pillow can be very helpful for support. If the plane has a headrest, keep the back of your head centred on it. Some headrests will bend up at the sides to support your head.

If you are reading, try to bring the book/magazine up towards your head and look down with your eyes without bending your neck.

Keep shifting your weight to avoid pressure points.

Try to maintain an angle of 90 degrees at your hips, knees and elbows by repositioning your arm rests and seat if possible.

If you are on a plane or train, stretch and go for a walk up the aisle as often as you can. If you are in a car, stop for regular breaks every hour or so.

Pump your feet and ankles up and down and circle them frequently. This is good for your circulation and helps prevent blood clots.

Drink plenty of water.

If you are talking to someone beside you, try not to twist your body towards them. Rather, turn your head.

Some deep breathing every hour or so is beneficial to your lungs, circulation and overall relaxation, especially if you encounter turbulence. Breathe and relax through it, if you can!

REFERENCES

1. Freburger J. K., Holmes G. M., Agans R. P., Jackman A. M., Darter J. D., Wallace A. S., Castel L. D., Kalsbeek W. D., Carey T. S.,
   Feb. 2009. "The Rising Prevalance of Chronic Low Back Pain", Archives Internal Medicine, American Medical Association, vol. 169 No. 3, pp. 251 - 258.

2. Kirkley A., Birmingham T. B., Litchfield R.B., Giffin J. R., Willits K. R., Wong C. J., Feagan B. G., Donner A., Griffin S. H., D'Ascanio L. M., Pope J. E., Fowler P. J.,
   Sept. 2008. "A Randomized Trial of Arthroscopic Surgery for Osteoarthritis of the Knee",
   The New England Journal of Medicine, vol. 359, No. 11.

3. National Health Service (NHS) website, Oct 2011, "Back Pain - Overview - Back Pain", http://www.nhs.uk/Conditions/Back-pain/Pages/Introduction.aspx.

4. National Health Service (NHS) website, Oct 2011, "Back Pain - Overview - Preventing Back Pain", http://www.nhs.uk/Conditions/Back-pain/Pages/Prevention.aspx.

5. Horowitz S., Aug. 2010, "Health Benefits of Meditation: What the Newest Research Shows", Alternative and Complementary Therapies,
   vol.16, Issue 4, pp 223-228.

6. Spiegel K., Leproult R., Van Cauter E., Oct. 1999, "Impact of Sleep Debt on Metabolic and Endocrine Function", The Lancet, Elsevier, Vol. 354.

RESOURCES

The Use of The Self
F.M. Alexander

Live Better: Alexander Technique.
Exercises and Inspirations for Well-being.
By Joe Searby
ISBN number: 978-1-84483-389-4

Pilates
The complete Guide to Joseph H. Pilates
Techniques of physical Conditioning
By Allan Menezes

Simple/inexpensive, sit/stand furniture option for computer workers
Raising the Bar and Freeing the Spine blog. Sandrin Leung Design
http://www.sandrinleung.com/raising-the-bar-freeing-the-spine/

The Breast Feeding Pillow
"My Breast Friend"

Healthy Aging For Dummies
by Brent Agin MD and Sharon Perkins RN (Jan 10, 2008).

INDEX

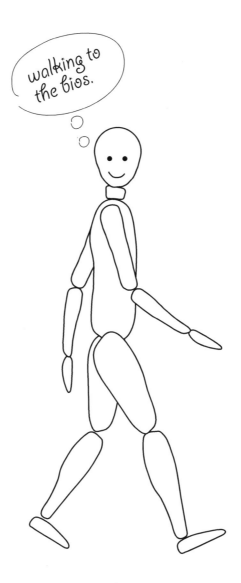

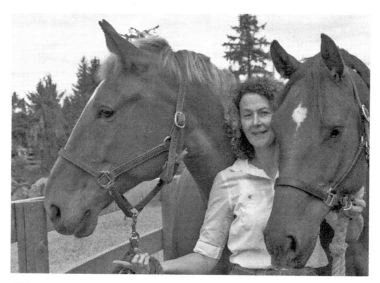

Photograph by Teresa Wyper

ROSALIND FERRY was born in Zimbabwe and grew up in Kenya, East Africa. Her father was a doctor specializing in tropical medicine and her mother a nurse. She had an adventurous upbringing, climbing Mt. Kilimanjaro, Africa's highest mountain, at the age of 17. Animals were her constant companions.

She wanted to be a physiotherapist from the age of 14 and did her physio training in London, England, and emigrated to Canada in 1972. She worked in hospitals in British Columbia and the Northwest Territories before starting up her own private practice.

Over the years, she noticed how the health of her patients and the time it took them to recover from injuries were greatly affected by the way they used their bodies ... and the harmony and balance with which they did so.

Her interest in posture and body realignment went hand in hand with her own equestrian interests. She found that the relaxation, awareness and balance required to ride horses was the same as that needed for efficiency of movement in almost all other pursuits. She also learned that animals themselves have a lot to teach us about the way we should move.

Married to a newspaper columnist, she has a son, granddaughter, grandson and two large horses. She currently lives in North Vancouver.

ELYSABETH BARNETT studied fine art at the Bath Academy of Arts in England. She lives in Toronto.

See more of her drawings at www.PWdrawings.ca

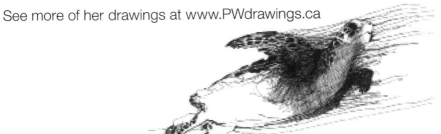

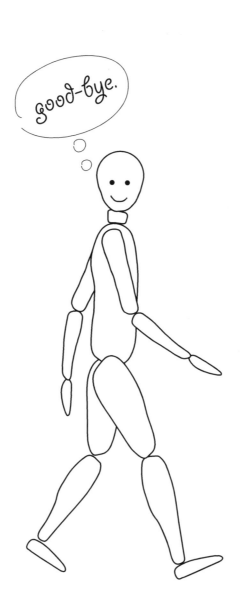